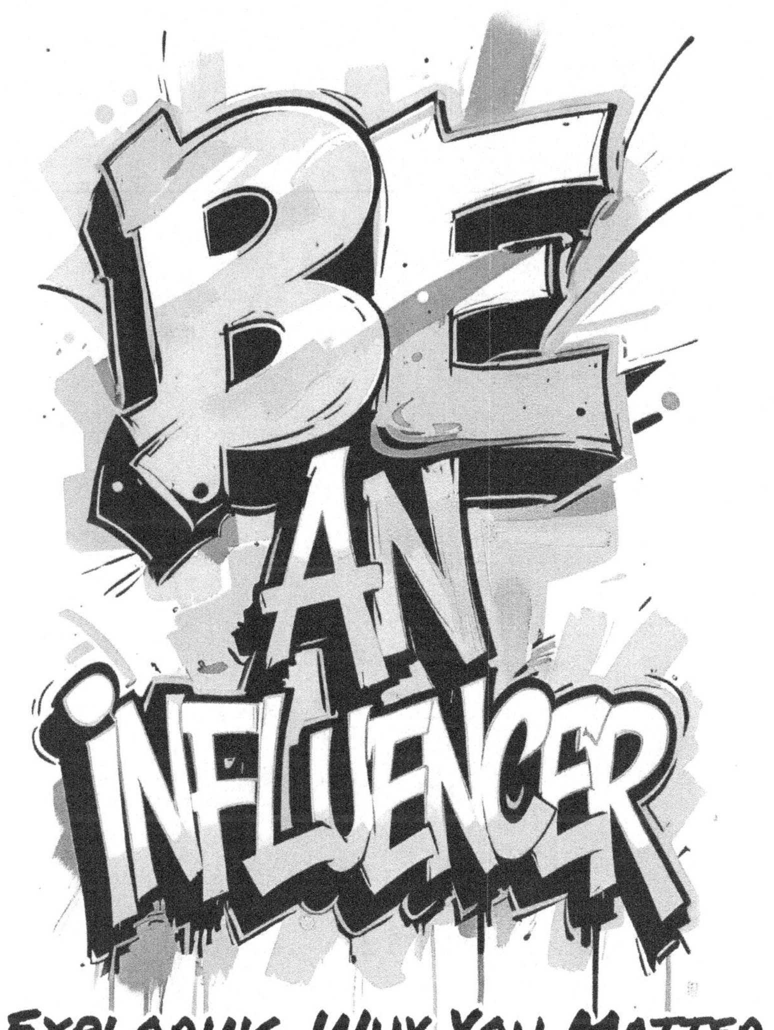

Exploring Why You Matter

By: Angela Stephens

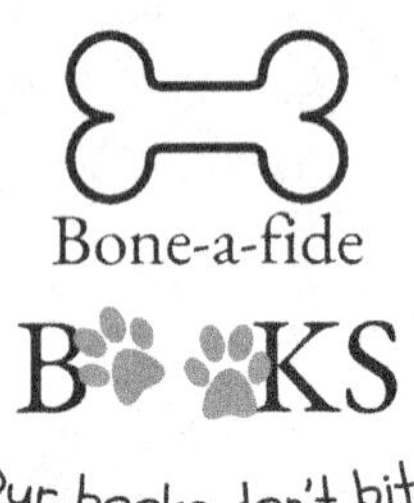

To request permissions, contact the publisher at ourbooksdontbite@gmail.com

Written by Angela Stephens
Graphic Design and Lead Editor Kandyce Valverde
Proofreader Kim Hunter

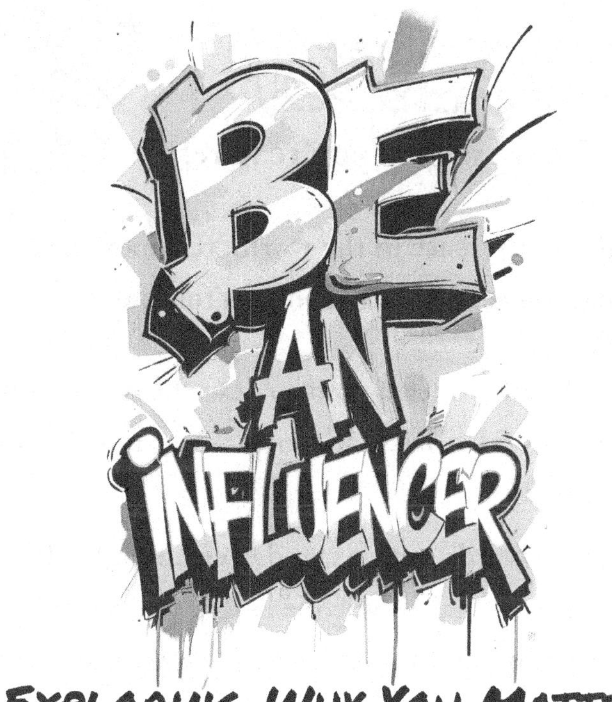

Exploring Why You Matter

By: Angela Stephens

WELCOME TO THE INFLUENCER PROJECT

We're so glad you're here!

Whether you want to make a difference in the world, feel more in control of your life, or simply figure out what's next in life, this book is for you.

The word "influencer" has become a term used to describe people with millions of followers on social media, famous celebrities, or sports icons, but the reality is far more powerful: *we are all influencers!*

Think about it. Our words, actions, and even thoughts have a profound effect. When we make someone laugh, we are an influencer. When wee choose to stand up for our friends, we are influencers. And when we live bt our values, we are influencers. Our emotions, ideas, and experiences all make us one of kind. Even the way we think about the world influences other people and maybe, just maybe. . .

THE MOST IMPORTANT PERSON YOU'LL EVER INFLUENCE IS YOURSELF.

Great influencers make a positive impact on others. To do this, they embrace what makes them different. They lean on their strengths and work on their weaknesses. Great influencers surround themselves with other great influencers and are not afraid to ask for help and get feedback to become better. Great influencers know that being great means making good decisions, building lasting relationships, and being intentional with who they are and who they want to be. Your journey starts now.

In these pages, we hope you will gain the knowledge to delve deep and develop the skills, confidence, and reflection to become the great influencer you were born to be.

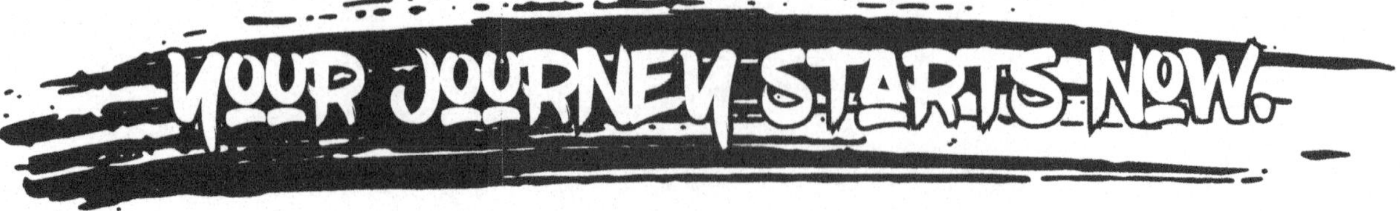

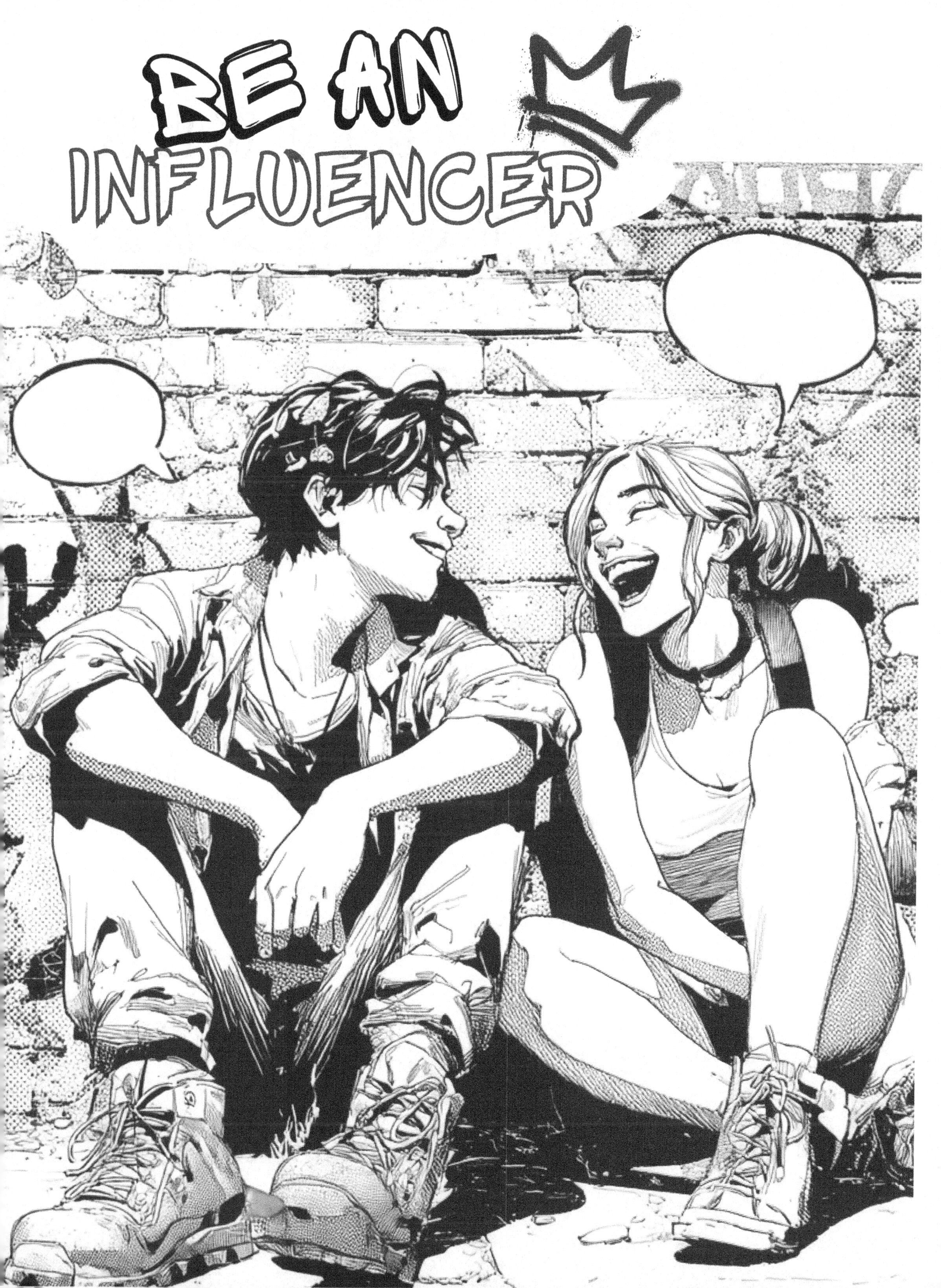
BE AN
INFLUENCER

A B C D E F G H I J K L M
N O P Q R S T U V W X Y Z

A B C D E F G h i J k l M
N O P Q R S T U V W X Y Z

Aa Bb Cc Dd Ee Ff Gg Hh Ii
Jj Kk Ll Mm Nn Oo Pp Qq
Rr Ss Tt Uu Vv Ww Xx Yy Zz

A B C D E F G H I J K L M
N O P Q R S T U V W X Y Z

Using any style of art or medium, draw your name on this page.

DISCOVERY JOURNAL

Section One: The Power of Influence 10

What influences you? 12

Influencer Quiz 13

My Influences 20

The Power of Environment 29

My Influence Map 34

The Dangers of Too Much Screen Time 41

Section Two: The Power of You 48

I Influence Myself and Others 50

The Me, Myself, and Why Treasure Map 57

Emotion Butterfly 67

The Emotional Decoder 73

Emotional Strengths and Weaknesses 75

Regulation Strategies 80

The Influence of Advertising 82

Section Three: Be an Influencer 90

The Power of Small Things 99

How do you Communicate? 103

Increase Your Influence 112

My Influencer Project 116

HEY THERE, INFLUENCER!

Welcome to "Be an Influencer: Why You Matter."

This isn't your typical journal. It's an interactive workbook designed to help you discover your own unique power to influence your life and the world around you. This journal is a safe space for you to explore your thoughts and feelings. There are no wrong answers here!

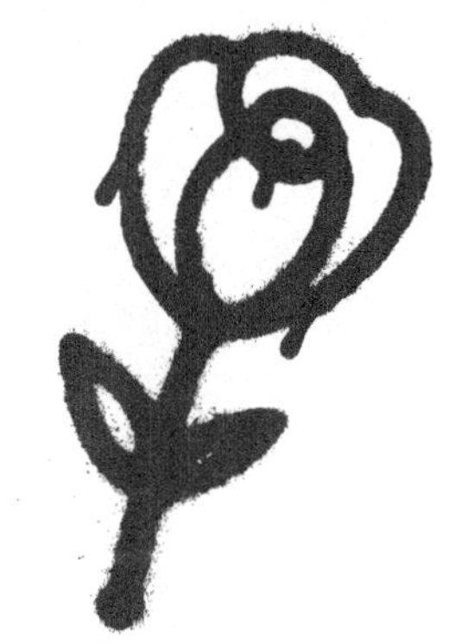

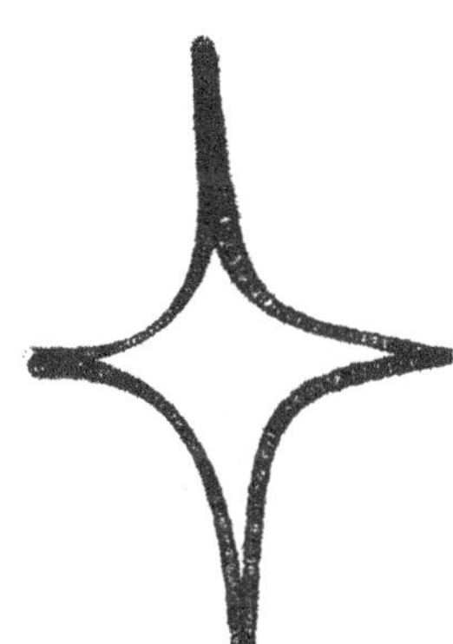

To get the most out of this journal, here are a few things to keep in mind:

- **Be Honest: The more honest you are with yourself, the more you'll get out of each activity.**
- **Be Curious: Don't be afraid to ask yourself tough questions.**
- **Be Creative: Use the space to draw, doodle, write, or whatever helps you express yourself.**

And remember, this journal is <u>YOURS</u>. So

WRITE IN IT

DRAW IN IT

OR JUST READ IT

Use it to find your own voice and become the best influencer you can be!

THE POWER OF INFLUENCE

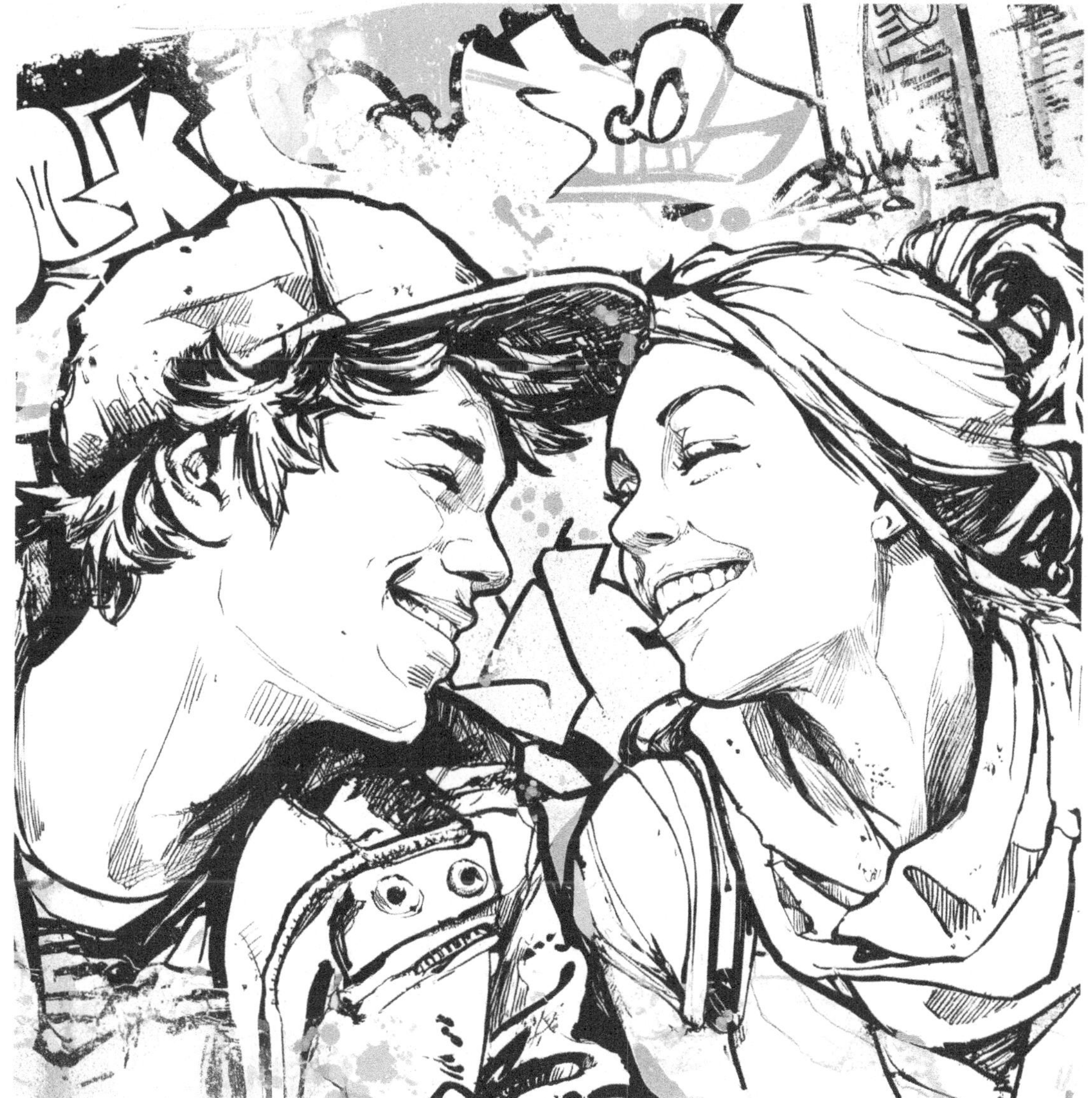

Your mind influences the key activity of the brain, which then influences everything, including perception, cognition, thoughts, feelings, and personal relationships; they're all a projection of you.

- Deepak Chopra

WHAT INFLUENCES YOU?

Look at the images below. What has the biggest influence on your life?

Rank the images from 1 to 6: 1 is the most important influence and 6 is the least.

Emotional Health

Intellectual Development

Popularity

Good Grades/Job

Good Conduct/Behavior

Focus

Physical Health

Skill Mastery

Relationships

Fame

Money

My Influences	What effect do these influences have on your choices?
1.	
2.	
3.	
4.	
5.	
6.	

QUIZ: WHAT MAKES SOMEONE A GOOD INFLUENCE?

Instructions: Circle where you fall on the scales below. Then add your responses up to find out which type of influencer you are.

1.What traits in an influencer do you look up to most?

1	2	3	4	5
making smart choices and staying focused	kindness and fair treatment	confidence and leadership	success and money	originality and self confidence

2. You are most likely to listen if a person...

1	2	3	4	5
gives good advice	cares about people	takes charge and inspires you	has already achieved big things	makes you think differently

3. A bad influencer is someone who...

1	2	3	4	5
encourages bad decisions	hurts or makes others feel small	uses power for selfish reasons	only cares about money	pretends to be someone they're not

4. You hope to help your friends be more...

1	2	3	4	5
smart and thoughtful	kind and trustworthy	brave and motivating	confident and capable	unique and real

5. If you could be known for one thing, it would be...

1	2	3	4	5
solving hard problems	making people feel seen	leading others	being successful	being creative

Quiz Results: Add your scores from the previous page.

0-7– The Boss

You are a natural leader with a clear understanding of what is right and wrong. People trust your judgment because you give great advice and value wisdom. You want what is best for other people and encourage everyone around you to make good decisions!

8-12 – The Giver

You have a talent for making people feel seen and cared about. Your friends and family deeply appreciate your kindness and the way you make them feel valued.

13-17 – The Hype

Confident and fun, you inspire other people to embrace life, take risks, and go for their goals. People bask in your energy, feel inspired by your courage, and trust you as someone they want to follow.

18-22– The Legacy

You value success, and know that money can bring freedom and comfort. You also know that to achieve great things takes work. This means you are willing to work hard because—you want your name to mean something and want your influence to last.

23-25 – The Vibester

You're authentic, funny, and unique. You don't need to follow trends because you create them, but that's not what really matters to you. You are focused on following your own values and living a life that is true to who you are and what you believe in.

What was your result? Did this surprise you?
What type of influencer do you aspire to be?

____

____

____

____

____

No One Like You

The slam of my locker echoed through the hall, but I was beyond caring. I threw my backpack over my shoulder and stormed through the long hall as quickly as I could. I kept my eyes low so no one would talk to me. I wasn't in the mood, especially since the quiz--the one I had studied for and still failed. That would have been bad enough, but at lunch, my best friend, Lisa, had snapped at me for not paying enough attention to her, and when I tried to defend myself, she was just gone. That hurt worse than any fight. And just when I thought this stupid day couldn't get any worse, the big, sticky Sprite disaster happened.

It wasn't my fault! The can just slipped. It tumbled from my hand so fast, and before I knew it, fizzing liquid had exploded all over the front of my jeans, making it look like I peed myself. Alex was staring right at me, watching the whole sticky, stupid thing. Whatever chance I had was gone. I jettisoned out the doors and down the steps, determined to get away from school as fast as I could.

But when I reached my front door, nothing got better. "So much for home sweet home," I thought, as the sound of my parents screaming at each other bled through the door.

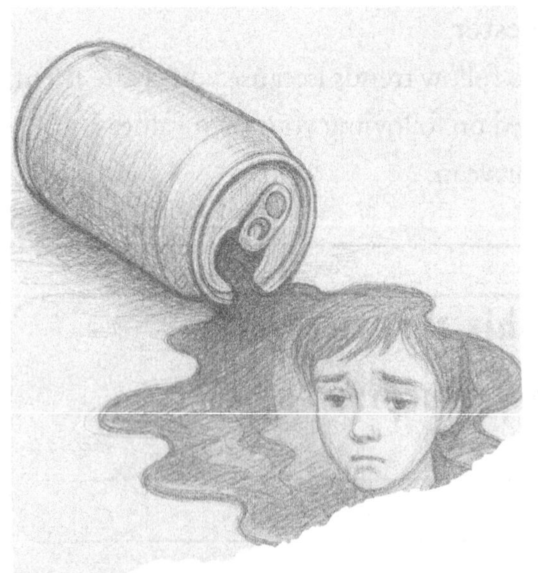

Money again. Always money. Well, that and the stuff I wasn't supposed to know about.

I sucked in a deep breath and crept through the door. Tiptoeing, I had almost succeeded in escaping the living room unnoticed when my eyes landed the framed photo of my baby brother. A deep sadness shook me as I forced myself to stop and look. The breath caught in my lungs, and I couldn't breath. He was so tiny. . . so innocent.

I clenched my fists and closed my eyes. I wanted to hate him for not living, to hate my parents for falling apart after he died. I already hated quizzes and school. . . and everything.

Suddenly, the yelling stopped. Worried they knew I was home, I rushed into my room, carefully shut the door, and threw myself on my bed. For a moment I lay there numb and unwilling to move. But then I opened my sketchbook, hoping to scribble out the pain.

I opened it to random page. On that exact page was a sticker my favorite teacher Mrs. Valverde had given me.

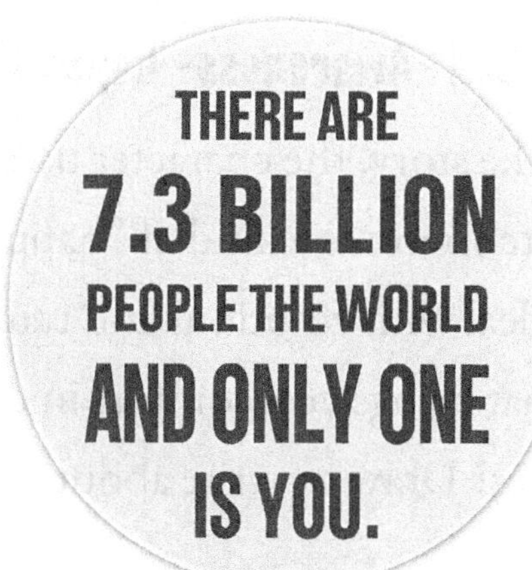

My finger traced the glossy paper as I remembered what she had said when she gave it to us.

"You are one of a kind. There will never be another person who gets to experience what you experience. No one will ever have the relationships you have." Her blue eyes teared up as she added, "No one can ever think about the world the way you do because no one can ever *be* you! And you have so much to add to this world, every day you are an influencer---so choose to be a good one."

That really hit me. My little brother's influence was so short. He had never had the chance to fail a quiz, to have a crush, or even a best friend. My stomach hurt. The fight with Lisa was so stupid. She was obviously hurting. But instead of reaching out, I was feeling sorry for myself.

"No one will ever have the relationships you have," Mrs. Valverde's words stuck with me. I hadn't even thought about what happened to Lisa today. What kind of friend was that? I picked up the phone and texted.

Hey, sorry about lunch. No excuses, but the quiz was a disaster. And I spilled Sprite all over my pants in front of ALEX and...please don't be mad at me

I held my breath, waiting for her response. It seemed to take forever, but then . . .

No way! My day was horrible too. Want to come over?

With one message, everything felt better.

Self-Awareness- Happy Place

In the story, the character uses their sketchbook as a kind of "happy place" to deal with emotions and trauma. What brings you comfort in difficult times? Draw or write about it.

What colors, sounds, and smells are in your happy place?

Who or what is in your happy place with you?

Impact on Others

The story says, "Every day you are an influencer—so choose to be a good one." How do you influence others?

Think of a time you influenced someone in a positive way. What did you say or do?

What is one small, positive action you can take this week to influence the world around you? (Example: smiling at someone, picking up litter, or being kind to a friend.)

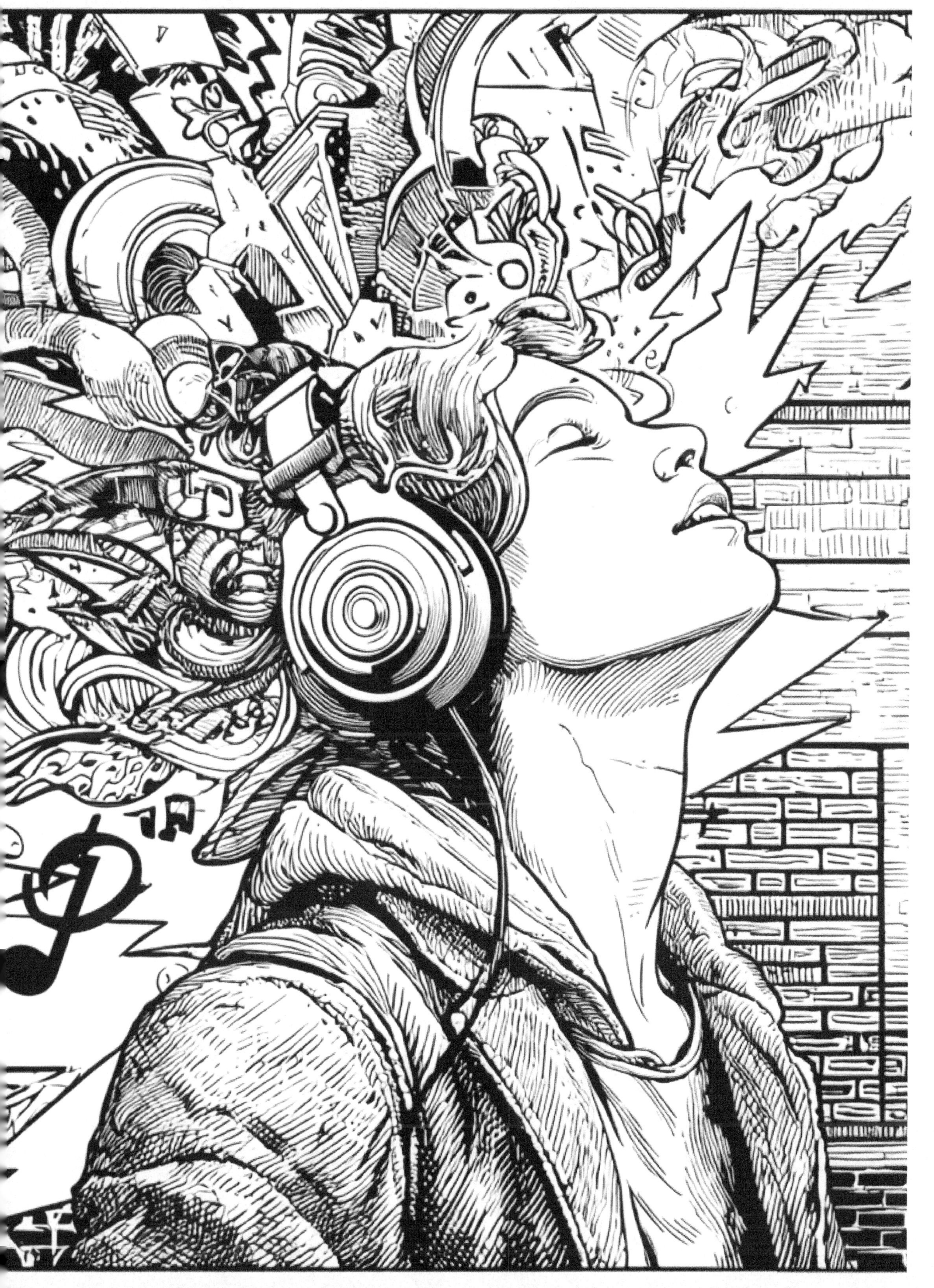

COLOR IT IN:
• Color the images that influence you
• Add doodles and sketches for images to the open circles
• Color the ones that influence you the most darker.

OUR SPACE INFLUENCES US

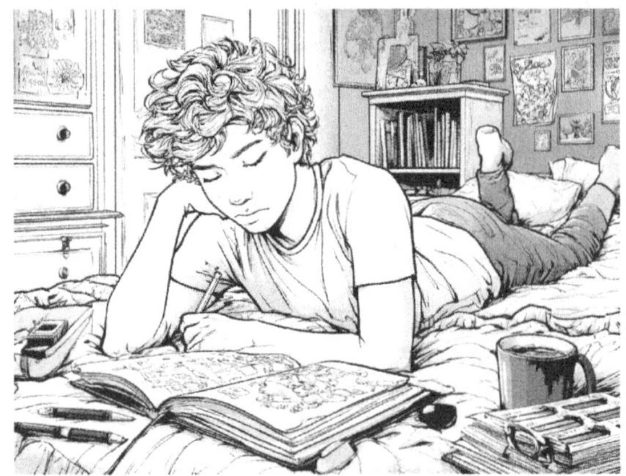

Ever wonder why you feel sleepy in a dim room or super energized when you're outside on a sunny day? It's not just in your head—your environment is secretly pulling a lot of the strings! Think of your brain as a super-powered computer and your environment as the software it's running.

Your brain is constantly taking in information from the world around you using your five senses: sight, sound, smell, taste, and touch. But it's not just a passive observer. This information triggers a chain reaction of chemical and electrical signals that directly influence how you feel and act.

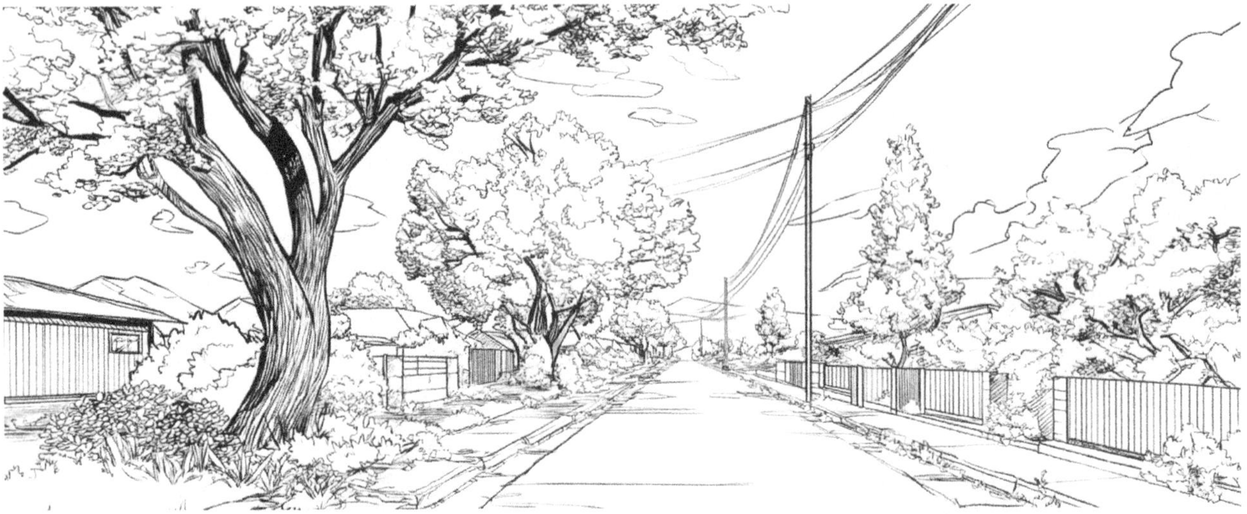

For example, when you see a clean, organized space, your brain releases "calm down" chemicals like serotonin, which helps you feel relaxed and focused. But if you walk into a messy, noisy room, your brain might send out cortisol, the "stress hormone," which can make you feel anxious or overwhelmed. It's like your brain gets grumpy and stressed out by clutter!

In the space below, write down five things in your environment that are causing you stress. Then decide if there is a better place to put them so they are no longer cluttering your thoughts.

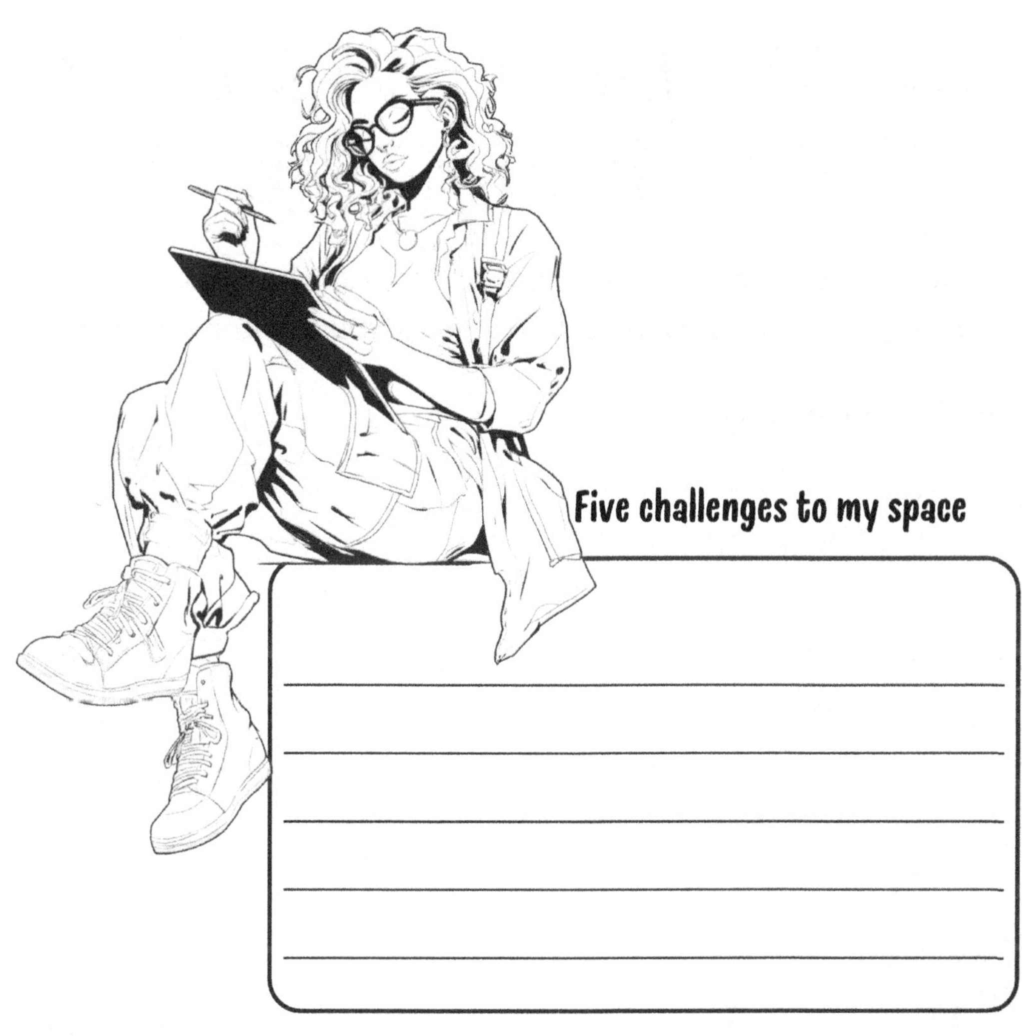

Five challenges to my space

What can you do about it?

MAKE YOUR SPACE MORE POSITIVE

You have more power than you think to make your own personal space a good place to be. Here are some easy things you can do to make your environment work for you

Declutter a little at a time

You don't have to clean your entire room at once. Just start with one small area, like your desk or a bookshelf. Getting rid of stuff you don't need can make your space feel bigger and less stressful.

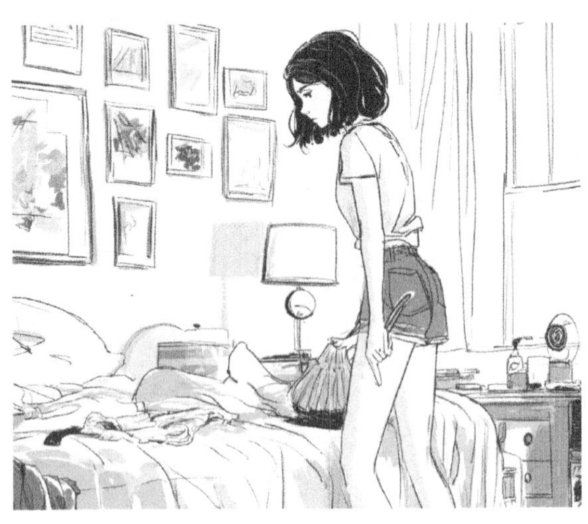

Control the noise

When you need to focus, use headphones to listen to calming music or just block out distracting sounds. This can help you concentrate on homework or a creative project.

Create a chill-out zone

Find a comfy chair or a corner in your room and make it your go-to spot for relaxing. This can be your safe space to read, draw, or just chill when you need a break.

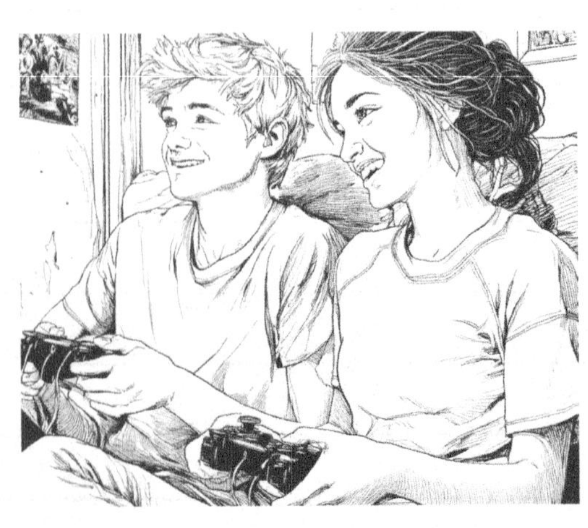

Add a touch of green

A small plant on your desk or windowsill can brighten up your space and improve the air you breathe.

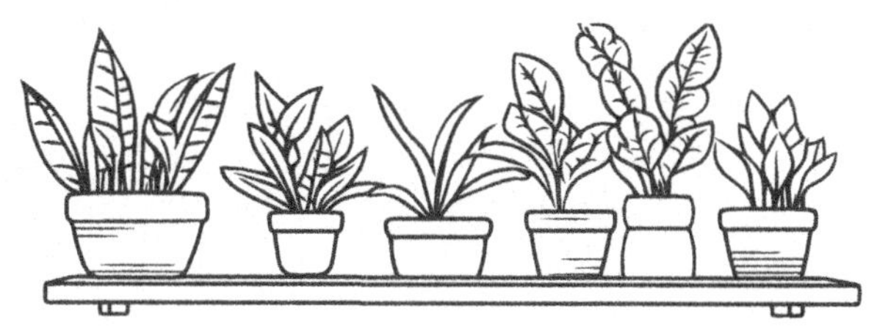

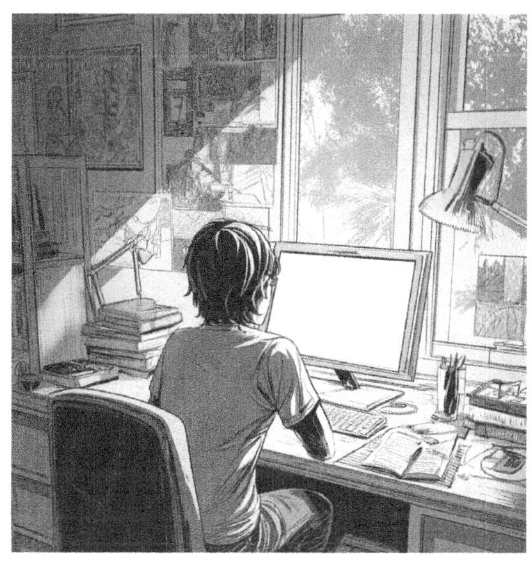

Let the light in

Open your blinds or curtains to let in natural light. Sunlight can boost your mood and help you feel more energized.

Make it "you"

Put up posters, photos, or your own art that make you happy. Surround yourself with things you love. It's your space—make it a place you enjoy being in!

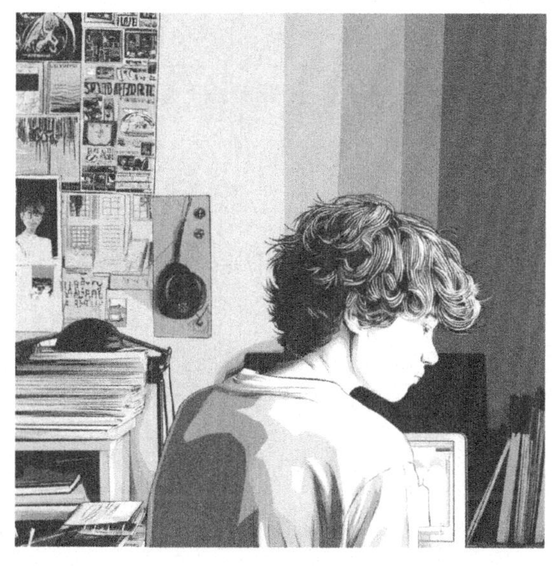

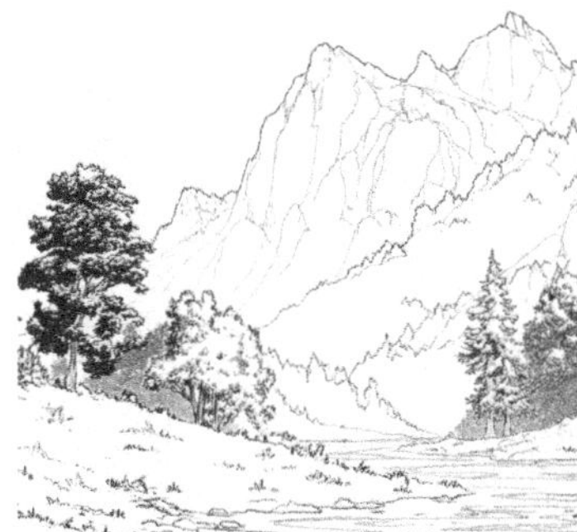

MY SAFE SPACE

Think of a place where you feel completely safe and at peace. It can be a real place (like your bedroom) or a made-up place (like a floating cloud). Draw it in the box below.

Add a "sensory map" to your illustration.

What do you see?
Label the colors, shapes, and textures.

What do you hear?
Add specific sounds, like music or animal sounds.

What do you smell?
Fresh rain, cookies baking, or something else?

What do you feel?
The temperature, the soft blanket, the cool grass under your feet?

When you're finished, look at your map. This is your personal blueprint for calm.

Whenever you feel a storm brewing inside you, close your eyes and return to this safe space you created.

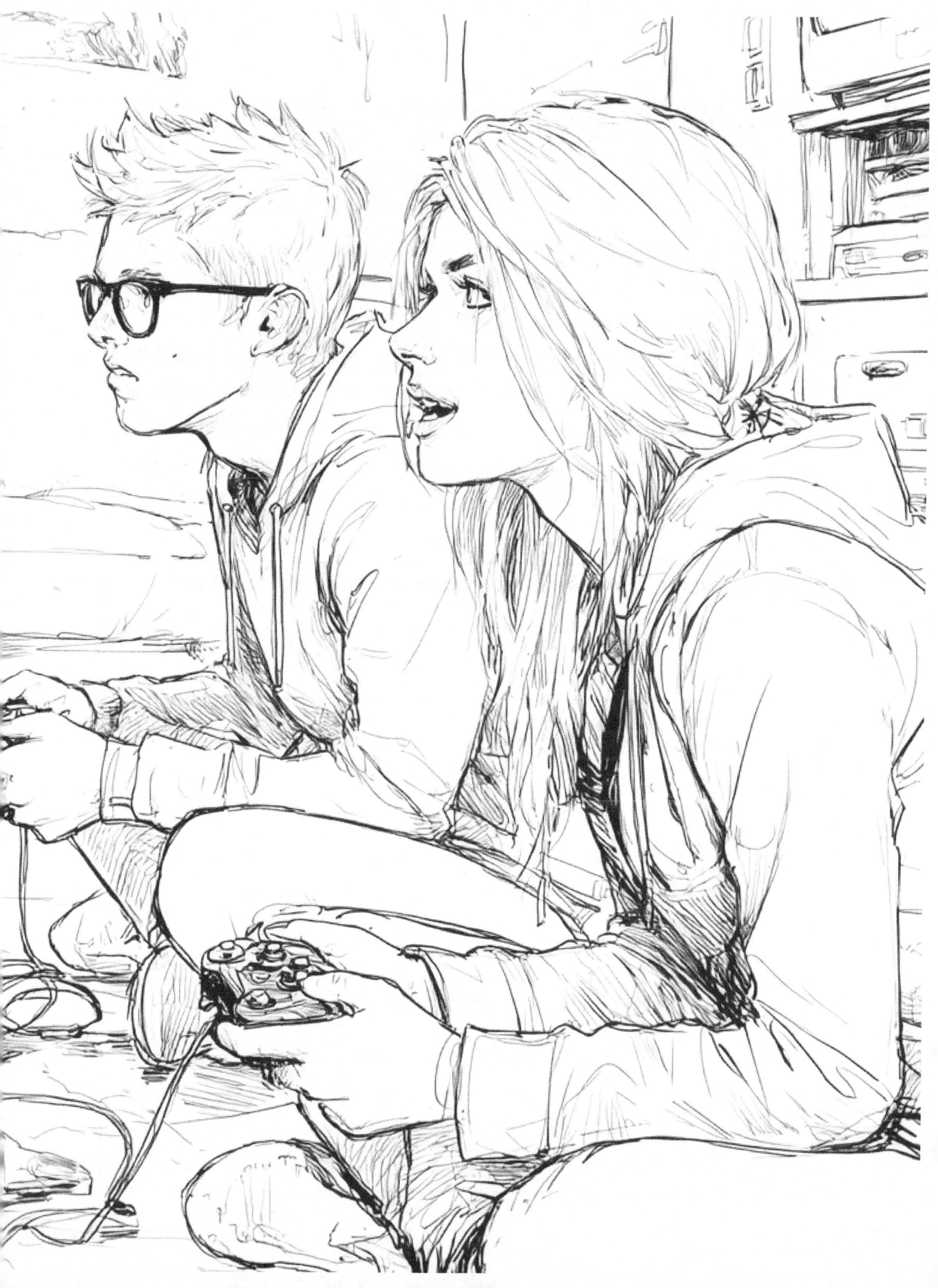

THE POWER OF YOUR ENVIRONMENT

LIGHT

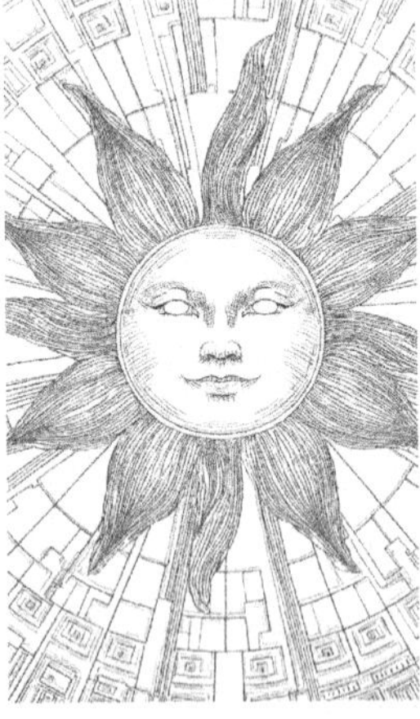

Light is a big deal! When your body gets enough natural sunlight, your brain releases serotonin. This chemical helps you stay awake. It also helps you feel happy. That's why being in a bright, sunny room can make you feel more alert and positive, while a dark room can make you feel tired. If you are having a hard time feeling positive, staying awake, or even being happy, then maybe it's time for a walk in the sunshine.

Did you know that 15 minutes of sunlight in the morning can help not only your mood but also keep you healthy ?

Let's get outside for some sun. What are your favorite outdoor activities?

____

____

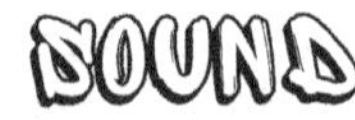

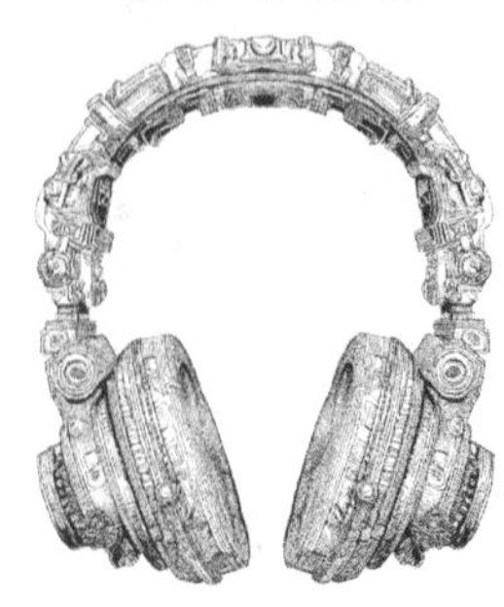

Ever notice how listening to your favorite song can instantly boost your mood? That's because sound waves trigger the release of dopamine. This is a "feel-good" chemical. When our bodies hear positive sounds, like birds chirping or waves crashing against the shoreline or gentle rain, we can often feel calm, relaxed, or even inspired. Music and sound can have transformative effects, so why not use it to your advantage?

Make a playlist of songs and sounds you can play to lift your mood.

____

____

____

____

CREATIVE CHALLENGE

My Mood Concert Poster

Imagine there's a concert where light and sound are the stars of the show. On your poster, draw or collage:

- The kind of light (bright sun, twinkling stars, neon lights, cozy lamps, etc.)
- The kind of sound (soft music, loud beats, birds singing, gentle rain, etc.)
- A title for your "show" that captures the feeling (for example: The Sunshine Symphony or The Thunder Jam)

NATURE

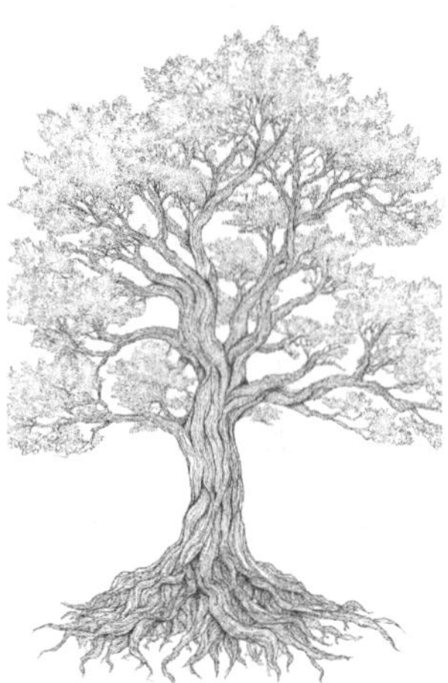

Have you ever noticed that when you are outside in nature, you can think better? Spending time outside is one of the best things you can do for your physical and mental health.

When we're in nature, our brains get a break from the constant busyness of screens and the buzz of modern life. It's like giving our brain a mini-vacation.

Did you know that spending time in nature improves focus, reduces stress, and even boosts creativity?

What natural sound (like rain, waves, or birdsong) brings you the most calm?

Let's go on a nature walk. Record what you experience in the space below.
What sounds do you hear?
What animals do you see?
What plants do you see?
What do you smell?
What does the air feel like?
What can you touch? How does it feel?
How do you feel after the nature walk?

CREATIVE CHALLENGE

My Mind Garden

Picture your mind as a garden. The natural, calming elements (trees, water, flowers, birds) represent focus, creativity, and peace. The clutter or "weeds" represent distractions and overwhelm.

Scientist call humans' need to connect with nature the biophilia hypothesis.

Draw, paint, or doodle this garden-scape—what's thriving, what's overgrown, and what might need tending or clearing out? Notice: what's the first thing you'd want to remove or nurture?

MY INFLUENCE MAP

Instructions:

1. Write your name in the square below.
2. Add the names of people you interact with regularly (friends, siblings, teammates, classmates, etc.) in the surrounding ovals. Draw arrows between you and others to show the direction of influence:
   - Two-way arrow = You influence each other
   - One-way arrow toward their name = You influence them
   - One-way arrow toward your name = They influence you

Optional: Use colored pencils or highlighters to categorize people:

- Blue = Someone who looks up to you
- Green = Someone you go to for advice
- Red = Someone who affects your mood a lot

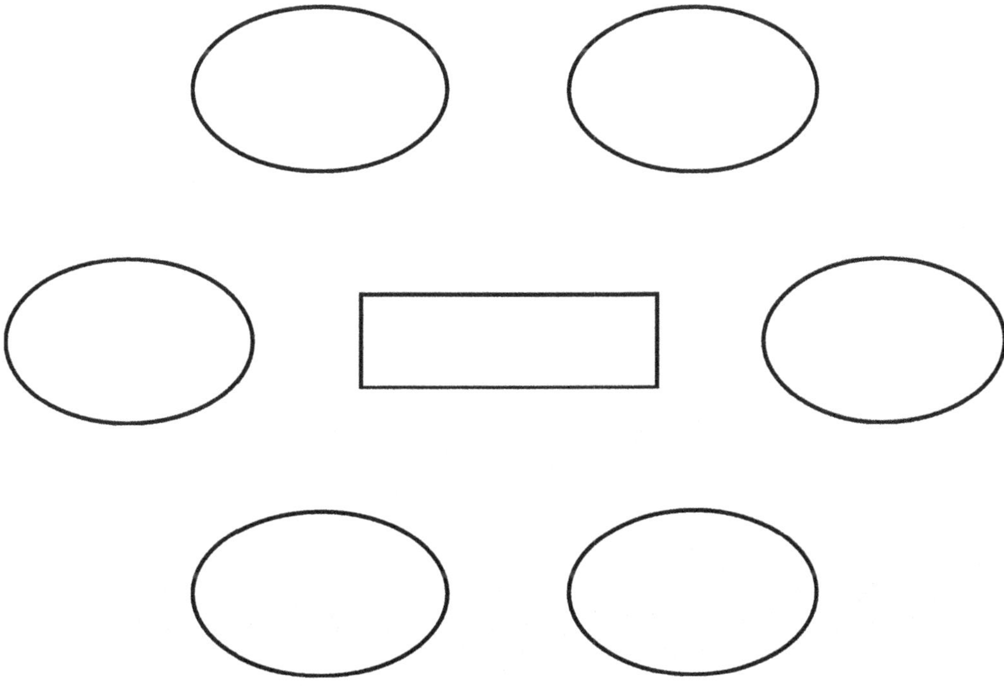

SKETCH BREAK

Positive vs Negative Influence

The friends we choose are a huge part of the influence in our lives. A great influencer is someone who builds others up, just like a strong bridge that connects people. They make us feel safe, supported, and valued, and they connect us to a better version of ourselves.

On the other hand, negative influences can make you feel insecure, small, or pressured. They act like a wall that separates you from your true self.

Your Task

Follow the prompts below to build a visual representation of positive and negative influences in your life. Use the blank space on the next page.

1. Draw a picture of a bridge. Underneath, write the names of two or three people who are a positive influence on you. Beside each name, write one reason why they help you be better.
2. Next, draw a picture of a wall. Write the names of one or two people who are a negative influence on you. Beside each name, write one way they make you feel less confident or happy.

Building good relationships is an important part of being a good influence because when you are a good friend, you are a positive influence, and you also attract positive influences into your life.

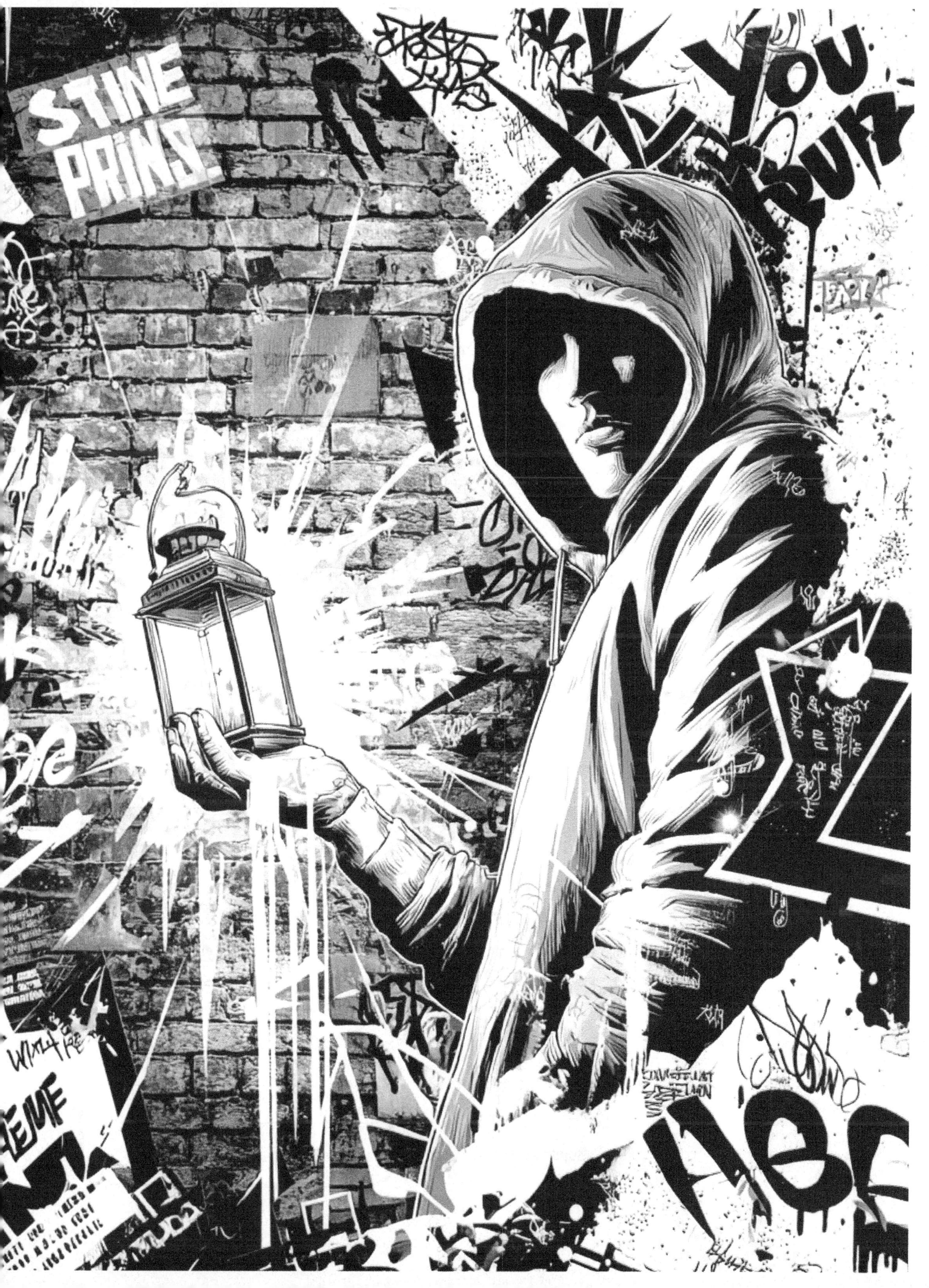
STINE PRINS.
YOU

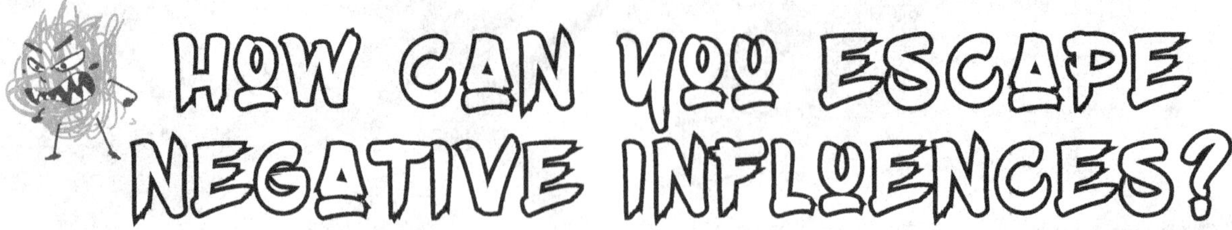

HOW CAN YOU ESCAPE NEGATIVE INFLUENCES?

Three Steps to Take Control:

1. Spot it: Recognize a negative influence. It might be a person who puts you down, or a media account that makes you feel bad about yourself, or a habit that you have.

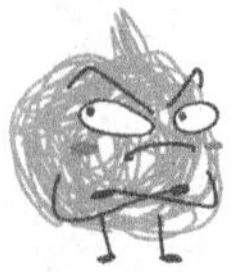

2. Protect yourself: You are in control of who and what you let into your life. It's okay to say "no." It's okay to walk away from a bad situation or unfollow an account that makes you feel bad. (It's good to ask a responsible adult for help)

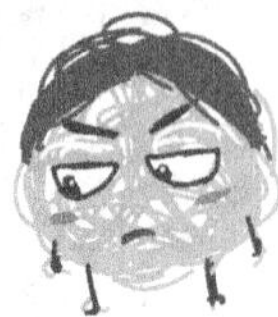

3. Find a positive replacement: Actively seek out good influences. Spend more time with friends who make you feel good. Find a podcast or a book that inspires you.

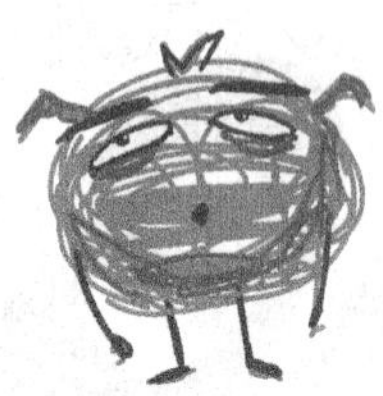

Your time and attention are valuable—take control and choose wisely.

Take control

Who is a negative influence in your life?

____

____

____

____

____

What will you do to protect yourself?

____

____

____

____

____

____

____

What good influence can you spend more time with?

____

____

____

____

____

YOU HOLD THE POWER

The Influence of Choice

Every single day, you your choices hold power. When you choose to watch a video, play a game, or spend time with a friend, you are choosing that over something else. These choices influence you more than you think.

When you click on a video, you are voting for it to be made again. When you play a game for hours, you are choosing that experience over practicing a hobby or talking to a family member. These choices build habits, and these habits build your life.

Write down the biggest influence and explain your feelings about it.

____

____

____

____

____

____

____

____

____

____

____

____

____

____

Think about the last two days. List all the things you chose to do for more than 30 minutes.

(Example: Playing video games, scrolling on social media, watching YouTube, talking to a friend.)

____

____

____

____

____

____

____

Look at your list.

Which of these choices influenced you the most?

Did they make you feel happy, stressed, inspired, or tired?

LISA'S EXPERIENCE

The Dangers of Too Much Screen Time

Lisa used to love to draw. Her sketchbook was her constant companion, filled with intricate doodles and colorful characters. But in eighth grade, a new world opened up on her phone: social media. Suddenly, her sketchbook sat forgotten under her bed. Hours that she once spent drawing were now spent scrolling through feeds, comparing her life to the polished, perfect photos of influencers.

While Lisa's feed looked perfect, her life was anything but. She stayed up too late, scrolling when she should be sleeping. And in the morning, she often woke up with a headache. Worse, she had a constant sense of anxiety that wouldn't go away.

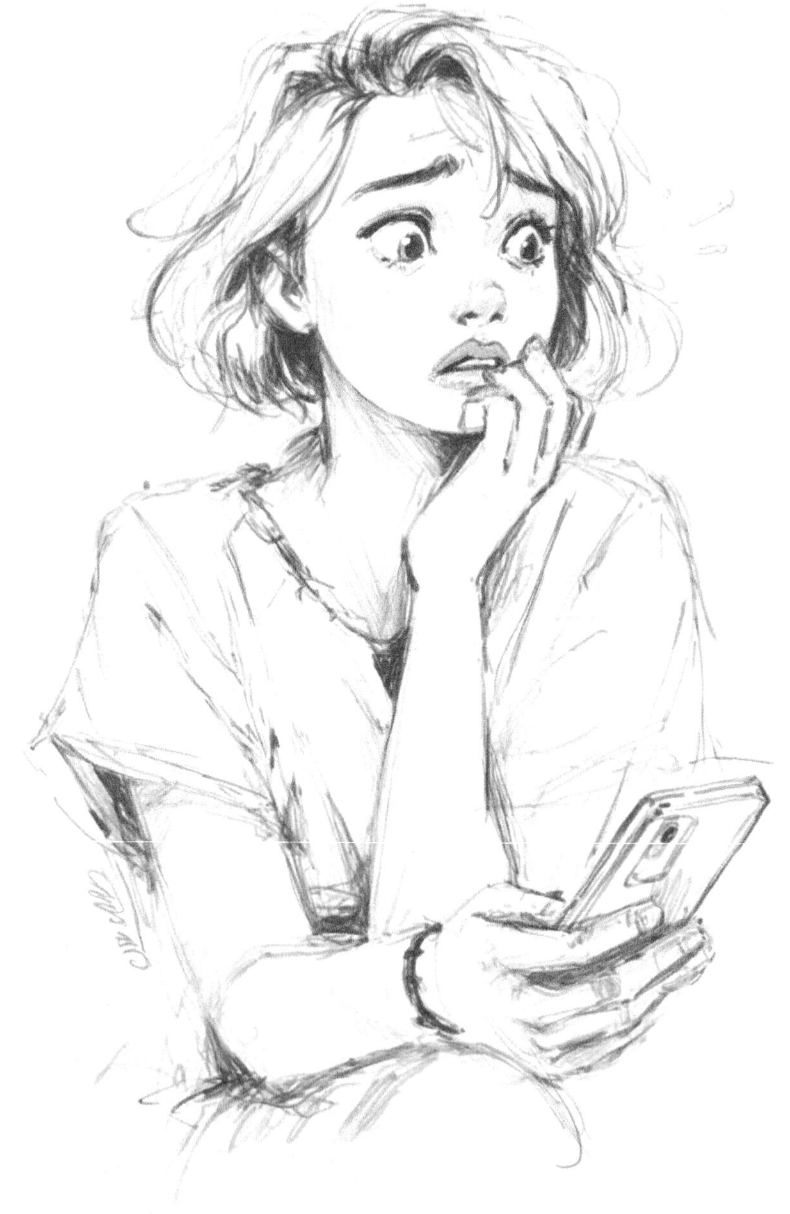

The more she scrolled, the more she felt like she wasn't pretty enough, not popular enough---not creative enough. Her love for drawing soon faded, replaced by a nagging feeling that she would never be enough.

Lisa's story is not unique. Social media can distort our reality, causing us to focus on what we are not, instead of what we are and what we have.

THE DANGERS OF SOCIAL MEDIA

Studies show that high screen time increases the risk of depression and anxiety in adolescents. The journal Preventive Medicine Reports found that teens who spent five or more hours a day on electronic devices were 71% more likely to have at least one risk factor for suicide, such as depression or anxiety.

(Source: Twenge, J. M., et al. "Increases in Depressive Symptoms, Suicide-Related Outcomes, and Suicide Rates Among U.S. Adolescents After 2010 and Links to Increased New Media Screen Time." Clinical Psychological Science, 2018).

SLEEP DEPRIVATION

The blue light emitted from screens suppresses melatonin, leading to a reduction in both the quality and quantity of sleep. Lack of sleep is linked to poor academic performance, mood swings, and a weakened immune system.

(Source: Hysing, M., et al. "Screen time and sleep among adolescents: a systematic review of the literature." BMC Public Health, 2015).

SEDENTARY BEHAVIOR AND OBESITY

High screen time often means less time for physical activity. Sitting and scrolling contribute to key risk factors for obesity, heart disease, and other chronic health issues.

(Source: Stiglic, N., & Viner, R. M. "Effects of screen time on the health and well-being of children and adolescents: a systematic review of the literature." BMJ Open, 2019).

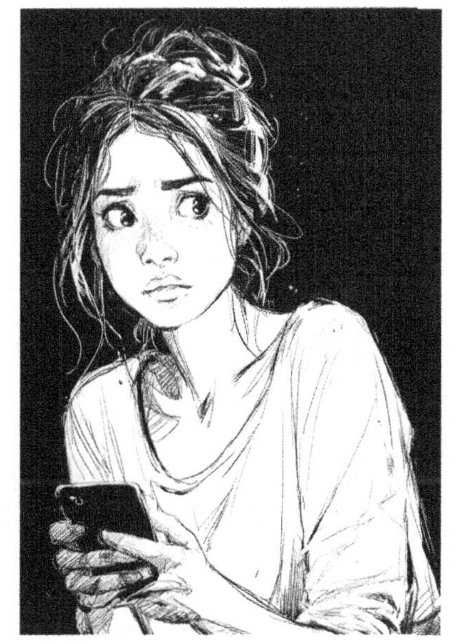

EYE STRAIN AND HEADACHES

Extended use of digital devices can lead to "computer vision syndrome." Symptoms include blurred vision, eye strain, dry eyes, and headaches, all of which affect concentration.

(Source: American Academy of Ophthalmology).

THE GREAT SCREEN TIME CHALLENGE

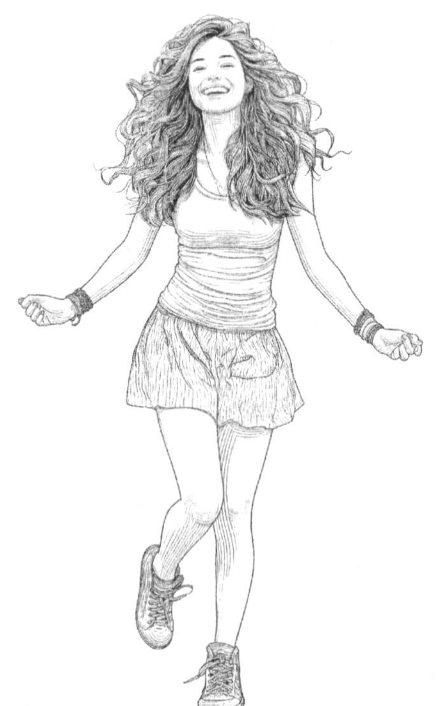

Welcome to the Screen Time Challenge! In a world full of glowing screens and endless content, it's easy to lose track of time. This challenge is all about becoming a super sleuth of your own screen habits. Let's dig in and figure out how to make your screen time work for you, not against you.

My Screen Time Tracker

For the next three days, you're going to be a detective, and your screen is your case. Every time you pick up your phone, tablet, or turn on the TV, mark it down. The goal isn't to be perfect, but to be honest. This is just for you to see what's really happening.

Day	Number of hours	Apps used	Why did you use it? (Were you bored, talking to a friend, doing homework, or for

Time to Reflect

What surprised you most about your screen time?

___

___

___

What do you think is a healthy amount of screen time for a day?

___

___

___

___

___

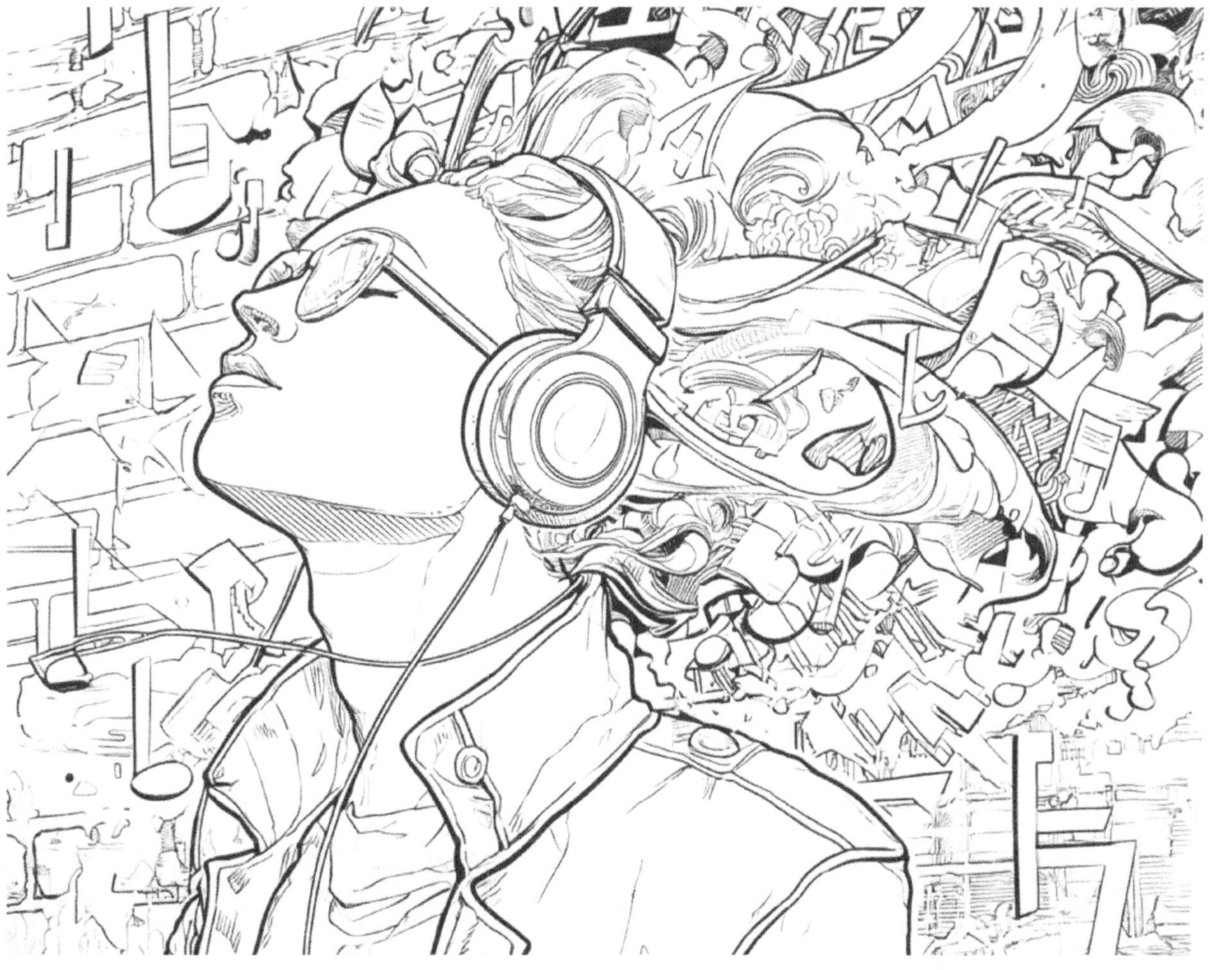

THE POWER OF LESS

Now that you've tracked your screen time and thought about who you follow, it's time to take control. This page is about finding a balance between the digital world and the real world. A little bit of screen time is great, but a lot can take away from all the other fun stuff life has to offer.

Think about some of your favorite influences and fill out the table below.

5 things you love to do that don't involve a screen.	
	3 people you want to spend more time with in person.
1 new hobby you'd like to try this month.	

It's your life, your time, and your attention. You get to decide what you give it to. Don't let your screen be the boss of you. Be the influencer of your own life.

PART TWO:

THE POWER OF YOU

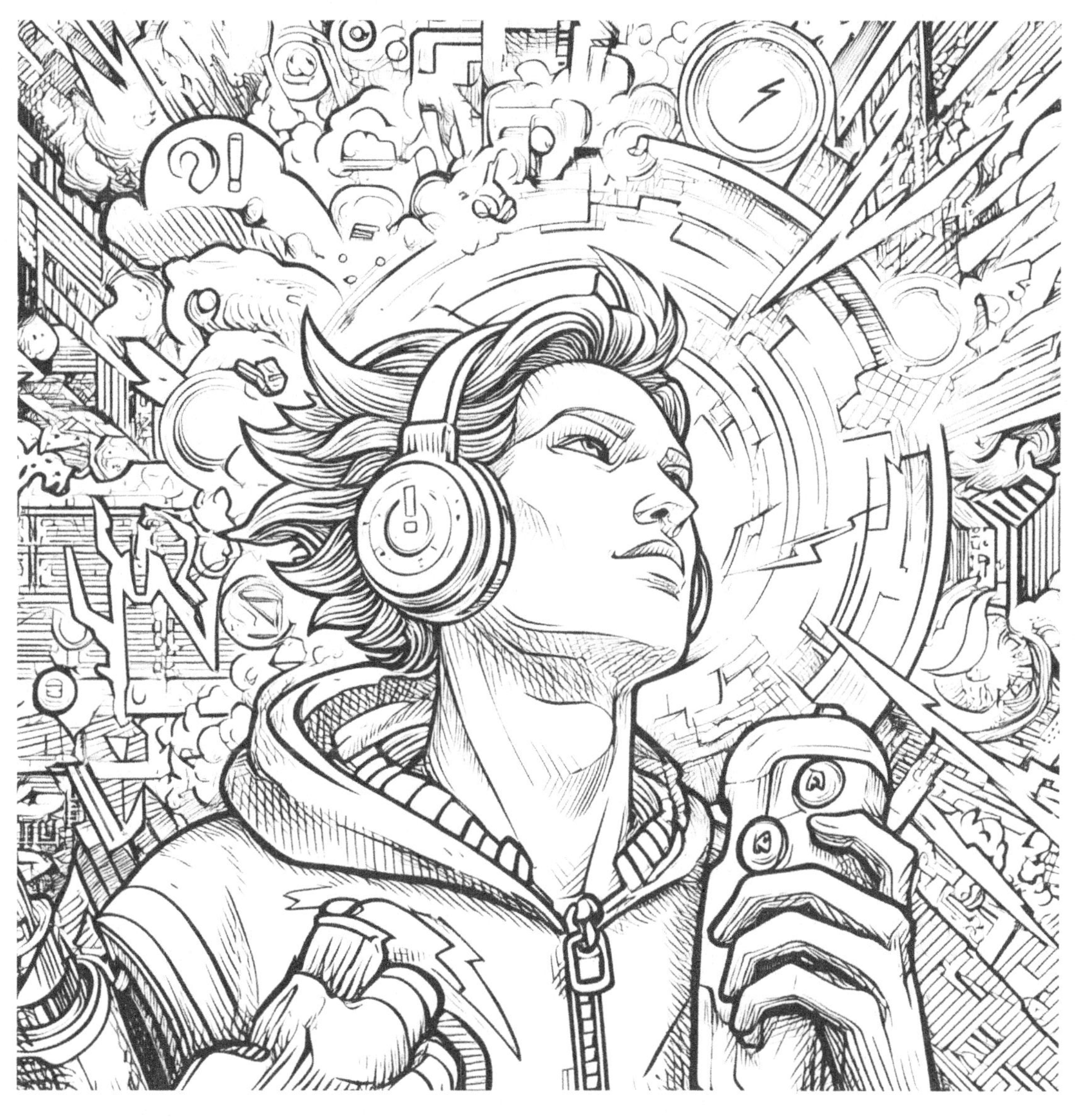

POSITIVE INFLUENCES MATTER

I INFLUENCE MYSELF & OTHERS

Brainstorming

Set a timer for three minutes. Write down everything about yourself that makes you you. Consider your hobbies, interests, values, personality traits, cultural background, talents, languages, and experiences.

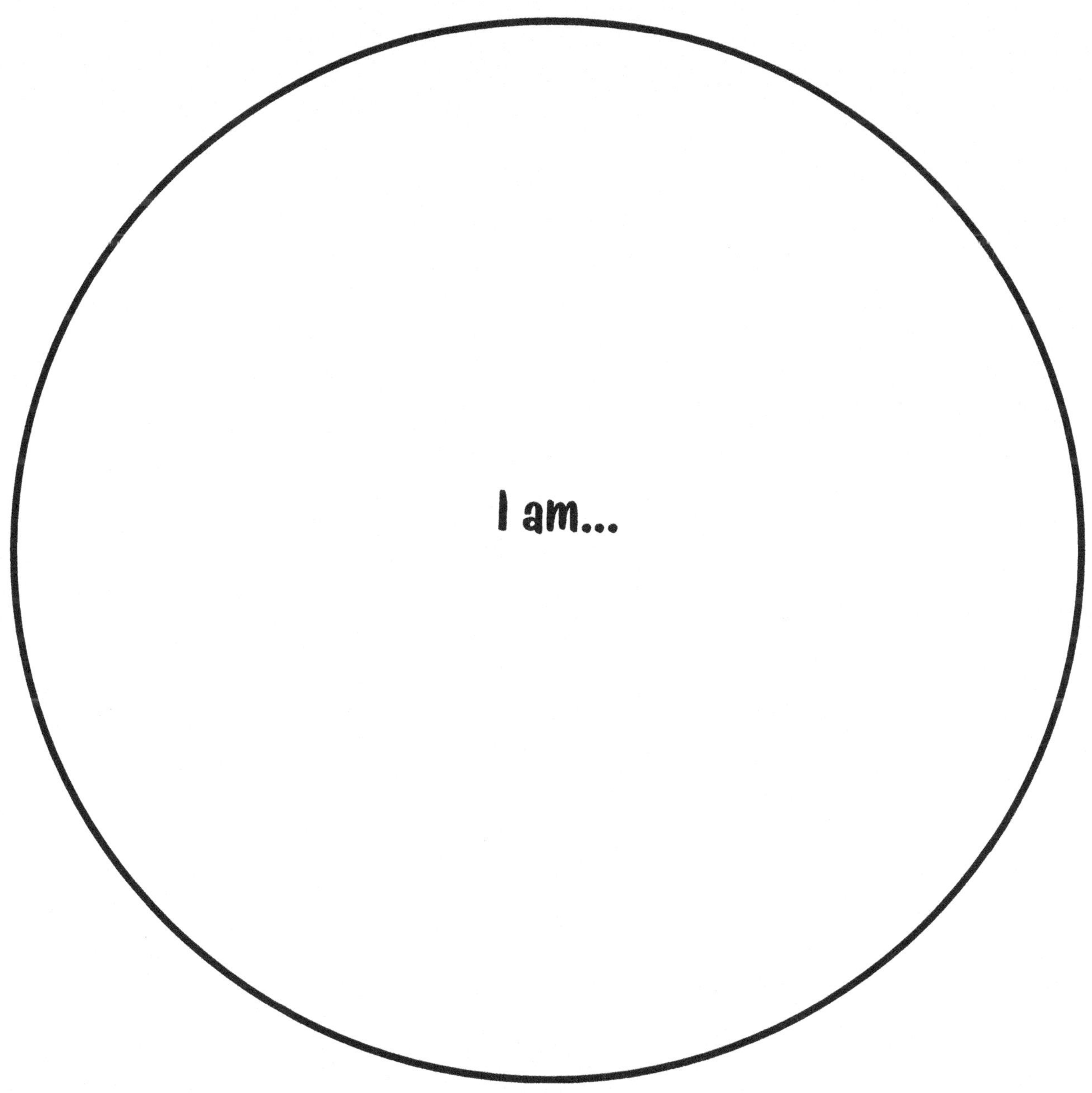

The most important person you influence is YOURSELF.

INTEREST INVENTORY

What interests you? Color in the top of the box of each item that you find interesting and have a friend color in the bottom to discover what interests you share. Use the key below.

Green: Yes, please! **Purple: Maybe** **Orange: It's not for me**

Reading	Soccer	Drawing	Dogs	Cooking	Music	Movies	Birds	Math
Bicycle	Playing an Instrument	Science	Collecting Something	Traveling	Shoes	Dancing	Camping	Nature
Writing Stories	Singing	Playing Board Games	Volunteerin g	Swimming	History	Photograph y	Acting	Shopping
Painting	Comedy	Football	Technology	Social Media	Hiking	Crafting	Cats	Speaking Another Language
Martial Arts	Superheroes	Baking	Making a YouTube Channel	Enjoys Sports	Trivia	Plushies	Reptiles	True Crime
Poetry	Coding	Pokemon	Fashion	Mythology	Enjoys fitness	Make Up	Jewelry Making	Road Trips
Card Games	Puzzles	Remote Control Toys	Yoga	Painting	Video Editing	Karaoke	Skiing/ Tubing	Fishing
Sewing	Rock Climbing	Debate	Memes	Architectur e	Basketball	Star Gazing	Anime	Chess
Video Games	Sculpting	Horror	Snorkeling	Volleyball	Journaling	Cosplay	Sleeping	Gardening
Ice Skating	Photograph y	Skateboarding	Meditation	Running	Horses	Mysteries	Animals	Baseball or Softball

SEEN & UNSEEN INFLUENCES

You're influenced by more than you realize. Let's figure it out.

"I Know"
Write the people, media, and things you know influence you.

"I Don't Always See"
Write influences you might not think about every day.

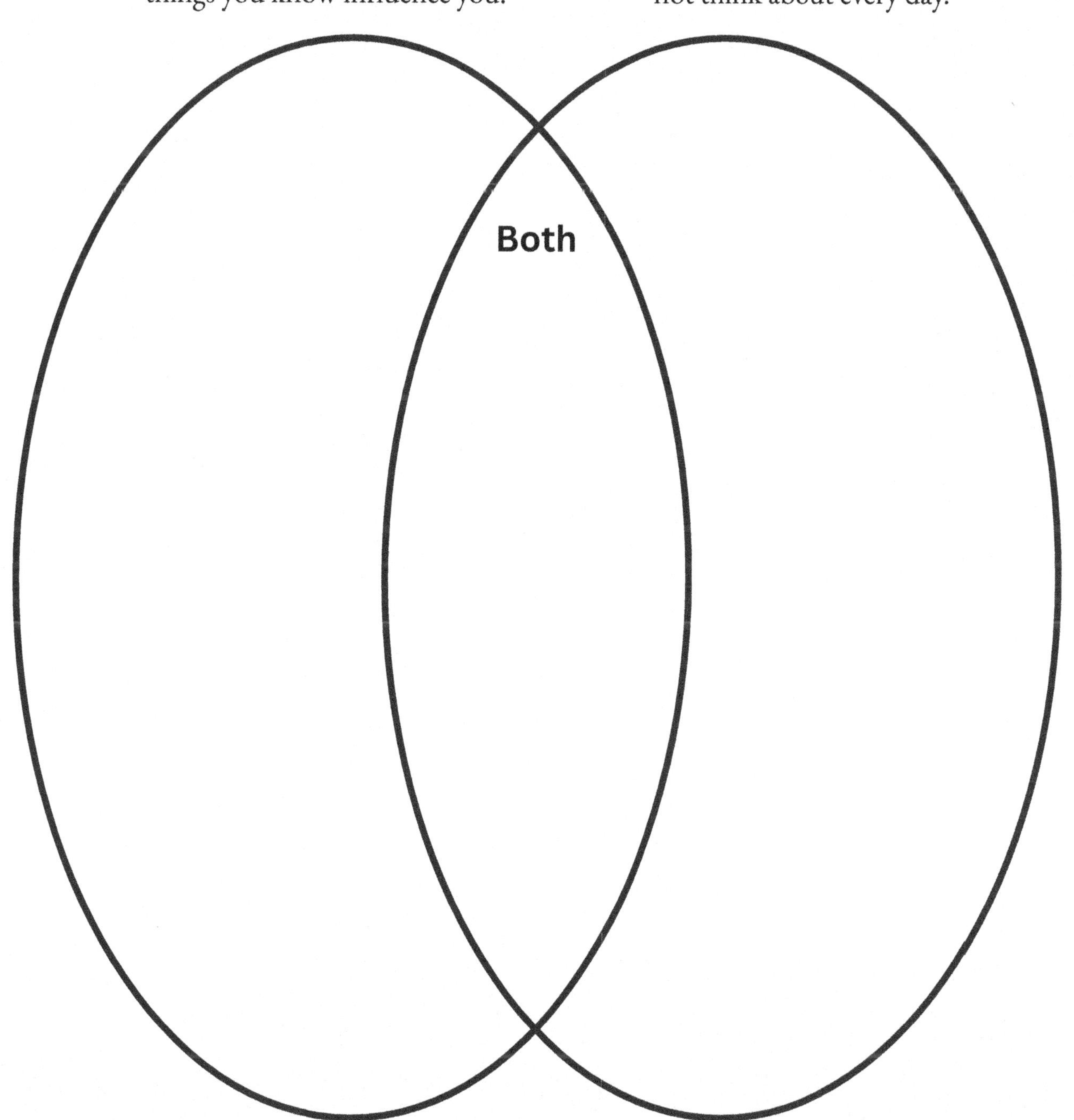

HOW DO INFLUENCERS IMPACT YOU?

Influencers can be awesome. They can teach you new skills, make you laugh, or introduce you to amazing ideas. But not every influencer is a good influence. Some might make you feel bad about yourself, or push you to buy things you don't need. It's up to you to decide if they are helping or hurting you.

Think about some of your favorite influencers and fill out the table below.

Influencer Name	What do they influence me to do?	How do they make me feel?	Are they a good influence for

Time to Reflect

What message do you often see from influencers that you wish you didn't?

What's the best thing you've ever learned from an influencer?

THE "ME, MYSELF, & WHY" TREASURE MAP

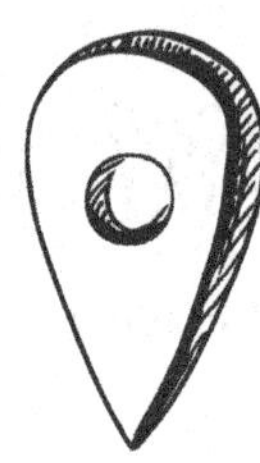

Now, it's time to get curious!

Pretend you're an explorer, and your personality is your treasure.

Ask questions to uncover the value of who you truly are

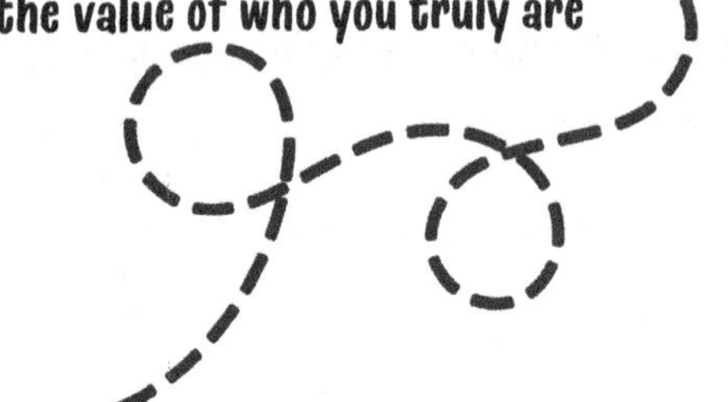

Gut Reaction

Who is a person (present or past) you admire or dislike?

Write down what you know about them and then ask yourself, "Why?"

What is it about their story that you connect with or react against?

Entertainment

If you were building a treasure box for your future self, what movie, video game, music, t-shirt, and/or books would you add?

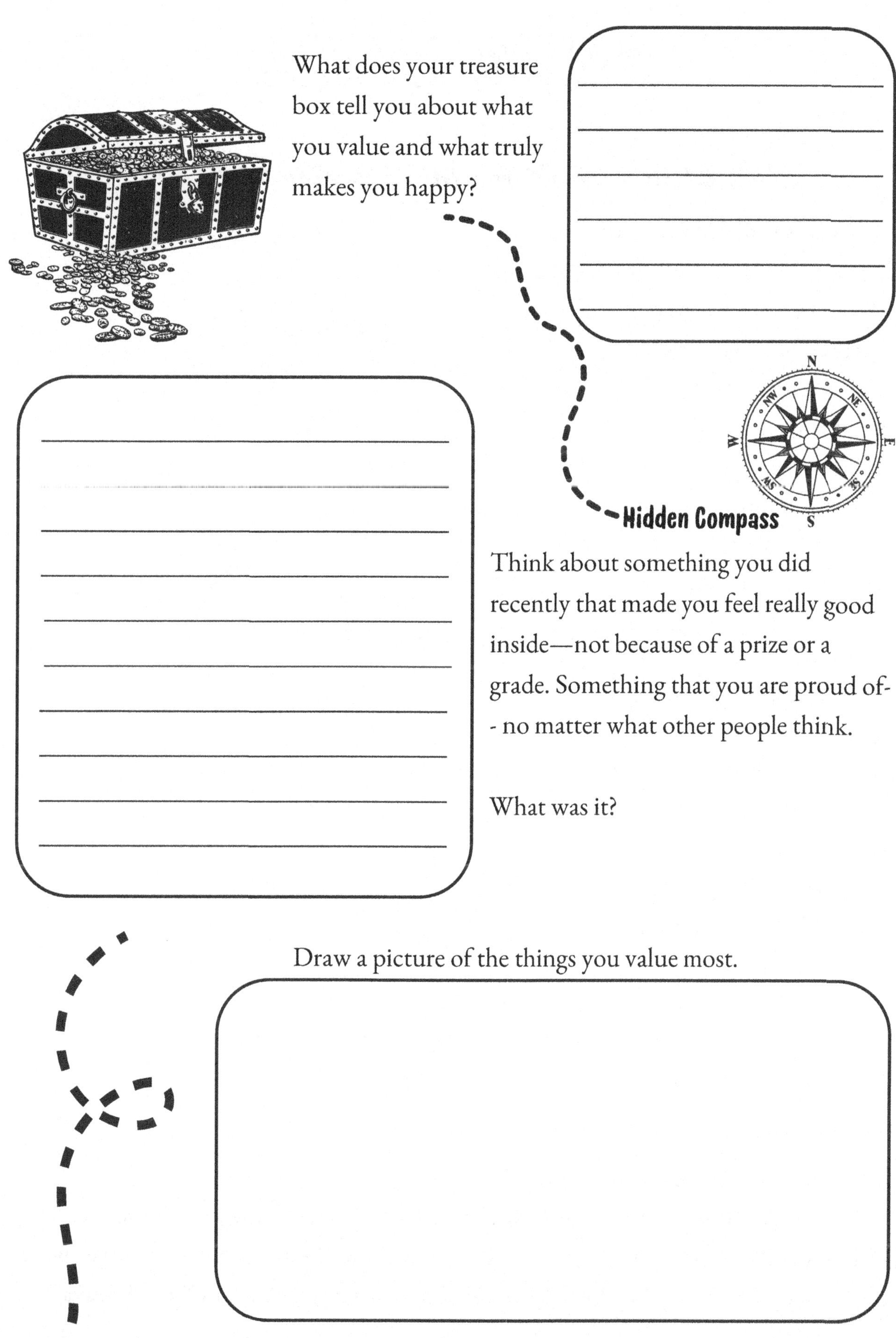

What does your treasure box tell you about what you value and what truly makes you happy?

Think about something you did recently that made you feel really good inside—not because of a prize or a grade. Something that you are proud of- - no matter what other people think.

What was it?

Draw a picture of the things you value most.

GOING VIRAL

The Ethics of Being an Influencer

Maya is OBSESSED with dance. Every day after school, she invents new routines and shares them online. Then one day, everything changed. One of her posts exploded.

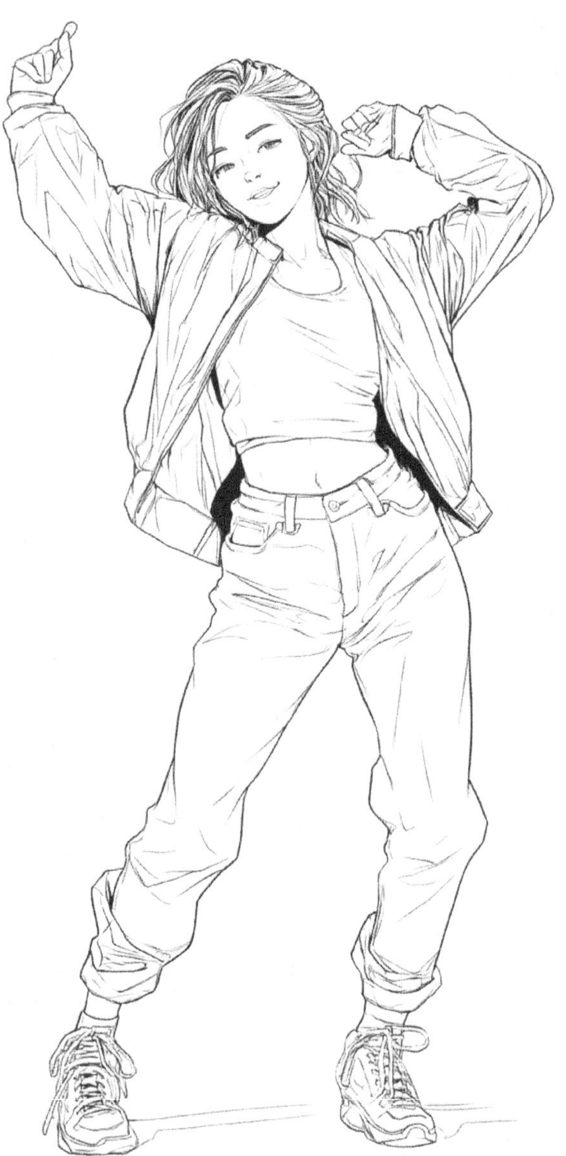

Within minutes, her BFF Liam called her excited. Within an hour, they had a thousand views--then ten thousand.

Overnight, the video went full viral with thousands, then hundreds of thousands of views. People were OBSESSED. Major dance accounts started sharing it. Suddenly, Maya was getting all the love–comments flooded in about how talented she was, and then people started copying HER dance! Maya had finally achieved her dream of becoming an influencer.

Then... everything changed.

A HUGE online celebrity, someone with millions of followers, who Maya adored, dropped their own video. As Maya watched, she felt sick. The moves were... suspiciously familiar. Like, beat-for-beat, step-for-step, an exact copy of Maya's original choreography. At first, Maya got excited, hoping the celeb would give her credit, but that never happened.

Instead, the internet went WILD. Everyone loved the dance! Some people immediately started calling out the celebrity dancer for stealing her moves. #JusticeForMaya started trending.

But the celeb's die-hard fans came out swinging. They accused Maya of trying to steal THEIR idol's fame. It gets nasty and fast. Maya's DMs were flooded with hate, and suddenly her incredible high turned into a nightmare.

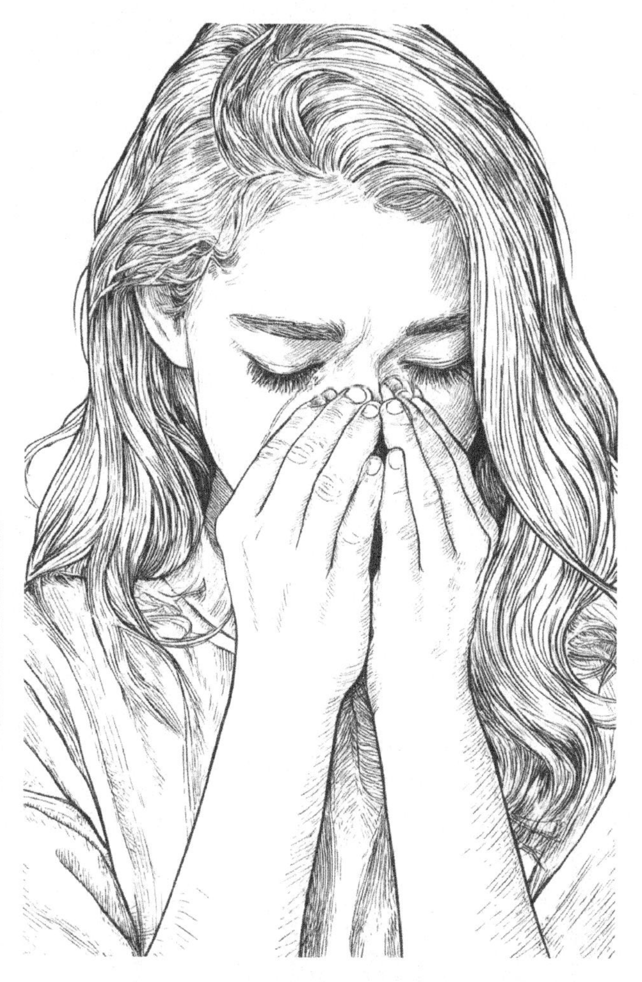

What would you do in this situation?

____

____

____

____

____

____

Circle whether you agree or disagree with each statement

Statement		
1. Maya was an influencer even before the video went viral.	AGREE	DISAGREE
2. The celebrity dancer had the right to use Maya's dance because it was already public on the internet.	AGREE	DISAGREE
3. Putting something online means it's free for everyone to take.	AGREE	DISAGREE
4. The other creators who stood up for Maya were the real heroes in this story.	AGREE	DISAGREE
5. Everyone in the story was an influencer because they all affected the way other people felt and behaved.	AGREE	DISAGREE

How can Maya use this experience to become a more authentic influencer, and what does that mean for her sense of self-awareness?

Influencer: an influencer is a person or group that has the power to change or shape others' thoughts, feelings, or actions.

Are some people more influential than others? If so, why do you think that is? Do you think the celebrity dancer or Maya was more influential in our story?

THE PERCEPTION PUZZLE

Which one of these stars looks different from the others?

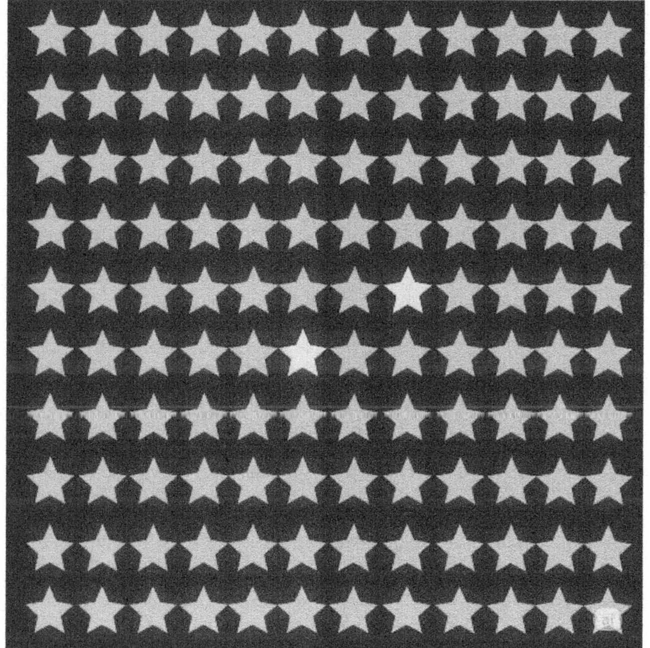

Did you find it right away? Sometimes, the answer is so obvious that we miss it. Our brains are wired to look for what we expect to see. Self-awareness is a lot like this puzzle: it's about training your brain to notice the things you normally miss about yourself.

What are two things that stand out about you?

____

____

____

____

Ask your friends or family members.

Find three other people who know you well and ask them what two things stand out about you. Write their responses in this space.

____

____

____

____

____

____

____

COLORING YOUR EMOTIONS

What color is your **Joy**? Is it bright yellow, like sunshine, or a soft, warm orange?

What color is your **Sadness**? Is it a deep, heavy blue, or a dull gray?

What color is your **Anger**? Is it a fiery red, or a dark, stormy purple?

What color is your **Calm**? Is it a light blue, or a soothing green?

What color is your **Anxiety**? Is it a swirling mix of colors, or a jittery black?

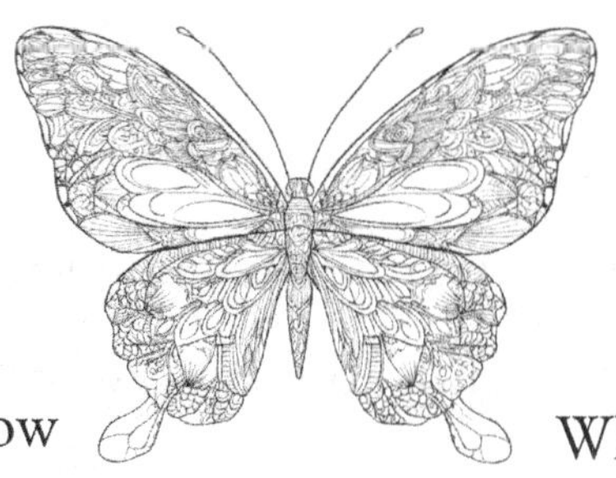

Color the words below with the colors you chose.

What do you think or feel with this emotion?

JOY	
SADNESS	
ANGER	
CALM	
ANXIETY	

Emotion Butterfly

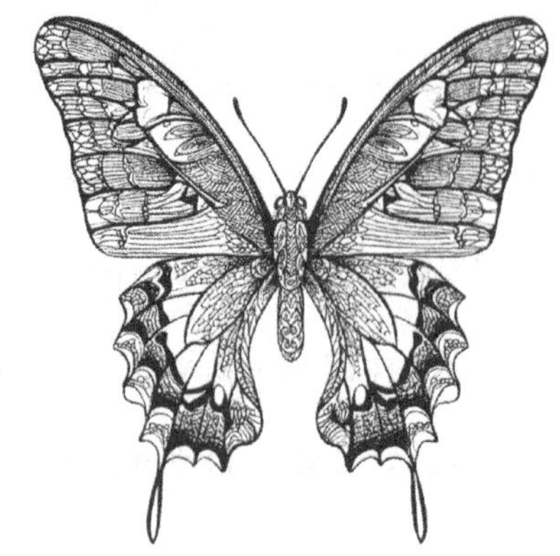

Emotions can make us feel all a flutter. They can change quickly and even color how we see the world. Like a butterfly's wings, our feelings are beautiful and powerful, and constantly shifting. The "Emotion Butterfly" is a first step toward understanding your own flight.

Imagine your emotions are like a butterfly's wings: sometimes they're a gentle flutter of joy, and sometimes a frantic buzz of anxiety. If you don't understand your emotions, you can be swept along, in a state of chaos, reacting to every gust of wind. This is what it feels like when emotions control you.

Self-awareness gives you the ability to let your emotions inform you, instead of control you. When you learn to recognize your emotional patterns, you will have a deeper understanding of who you really are. Emotions tell us when we are feeling anxious or sad. This information allows us to soar higher and find out why – only then can we address the root of the problem in a healthy way.

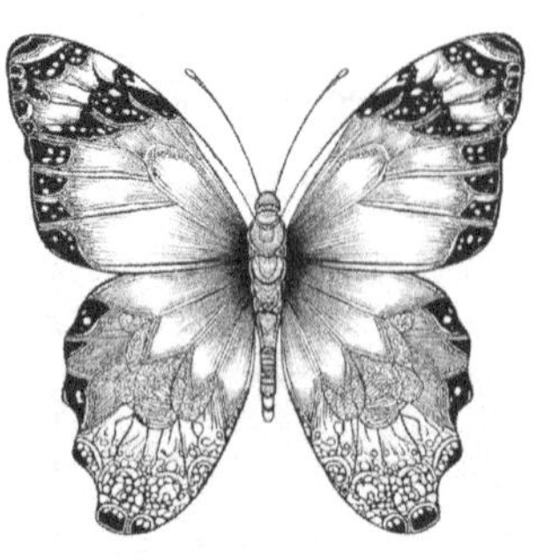

This is the very essence of being a positive influence. Great influencers do not chase trends; they make them. They do not flit off to the next big buzz, but contemplate the meaning behind it. The best influencers value their emotions, listen to their inner voice, and embrace their own unique emotional patterns.

Think about a time you felt your joy color. What were you doing?

Think about a time you felt your sadness color. What was happening?

How do the emotions in your emotion spectrum change throughout the week?

As you color the butterflies below, consider that every butterfly has its own unique wing patterns. Each with its own vibrant color patterns- just like you have your own emotional patterns. The more you know about your own emotional patterns, the more you can appreciate just how unique you are.

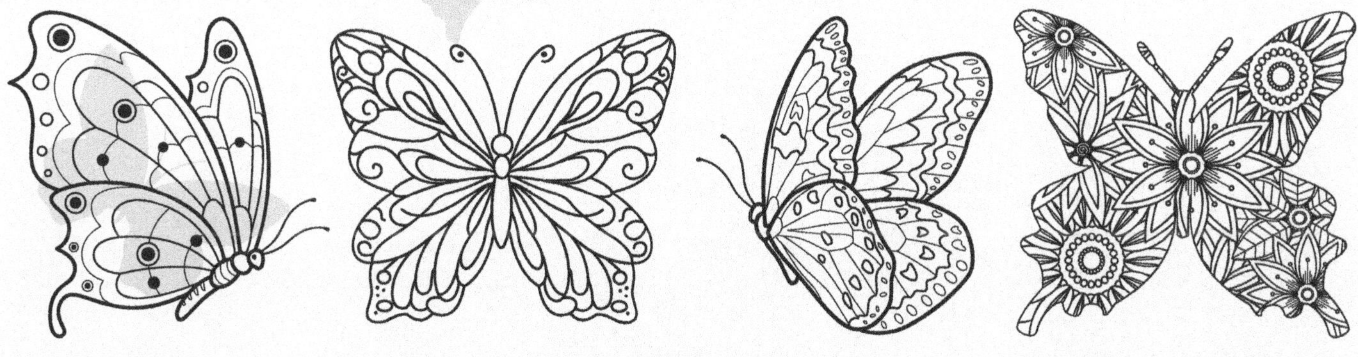

WHAT WOULD YOU DO?

This quick activity will help you notice your emotional patterns. Knowing your patterns is the first step toward being in control of your flight.

1 When a classmate makes a rude comment about your clothes, you most likely:

a. Try to act like you didn't hear them and just walk away. It's easier to just avoid conflict.

b. Immediately feel a flutter of anger and want to say something rude back or storm off.

c. Worry about what everyone else saw and wonder if you're dressed "wrong" in a desperate desire for belonging.

2 When you get a bad grade on a test, your first instinct is to:

a. Hide the test from your parents and try to forget it ever happened.

b. Get really frustrated and think, "This is so unfair!" or "I'm just not good at this!"

c. Post on social media about how hard the class is, hoping for some likes and sympathy.

3 When your friends are making a plan you don't really like, you tend to:

a. Quietly go along with it, even if you're not having fun, because it avoids drama.

b. Push hard for your own idea and get annoyed when others don't agree.

c. Change your opinion to match what they want to do so they will like you more.Your friend is feeling left out of a group.

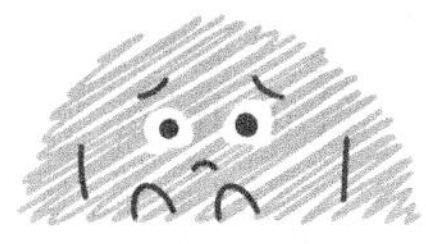

Your Wing Pattern

Count how many times you chose A, B, and C.

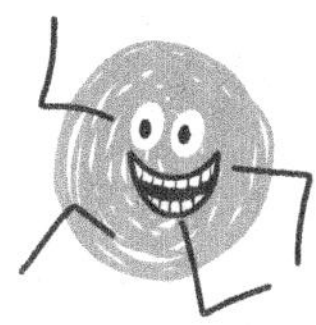

Mostly A's

The Hiding Butterfly. You tend to flutter away from conflict or discomfort. You believe it's safer to avoid and hide your feelings than to express them.

Mostly B's

The Stormy Butterfly. You tend to react to your emotions immediately and intensely. Your feelings can change quickly and feel out of control, like a storm.

Mostly Cs

The People-Pleasing Butterfly. You are very aware of what others are doing. You are quick to change your flight to match the crowd, even if it goes against what your heart wants.

THE EMOTIONAL DECODER

Understand your feelings so they don't run the show. Self-aware people know how to listen to their emotions without letting those feelings make all the decisions. They pause and ask questions that help them regulate their emotions. Use this chart to keep your feelings in check so you control them and they don't control you.

Core Emotion		It might feel like...	Ask yourself...
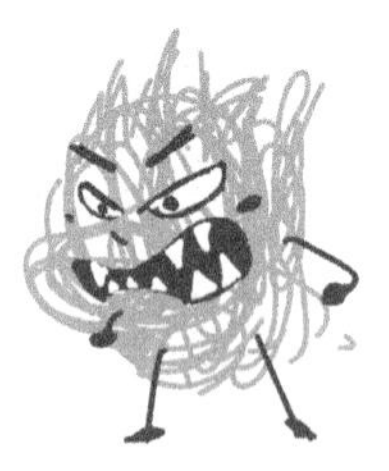	ANGER	Tight chest, tense jaw, hot face, fast heartbeat, wanting to yell	Am I reacting to what's happening now, or something old? Can I cool down before I act?
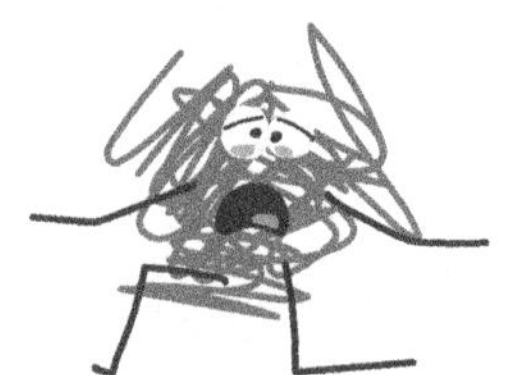	Sadness	Heavy body, low energy, quiet, teary, wanting to be alone	Is this feeling telling me I lost something important?
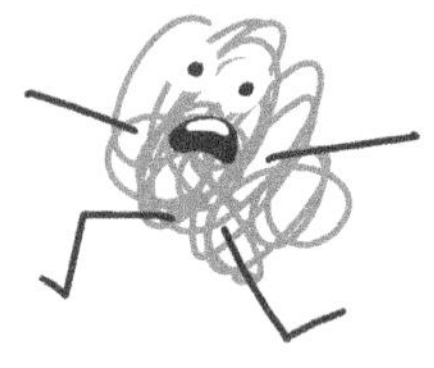	FEAR	Fast breathing, tense stomach, sweaty hands, wanting to escape.	Is this a real danger or just a "what if"? Do I need more facts before deciding?
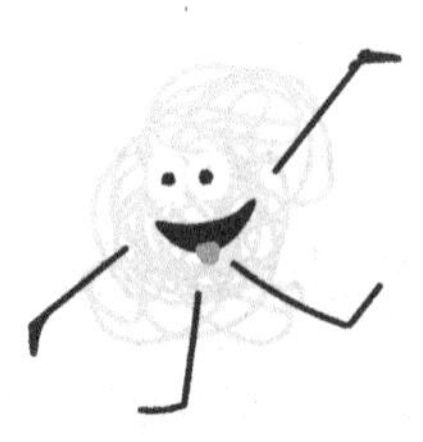	EXCITEMENT /ELATION	Light body, racing thoughts, big smile, restless energy	Am I making a choice too quickly because I'm hyped? Should I wait before committing?

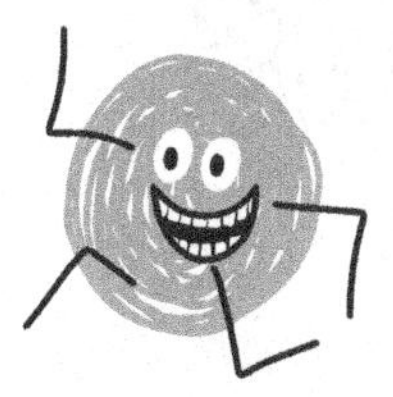	*Joy*	Relaxed muscles, easy breathing, smiling, calm energy	Is this something I can repeat or share? Can I enjoy it without rushing?
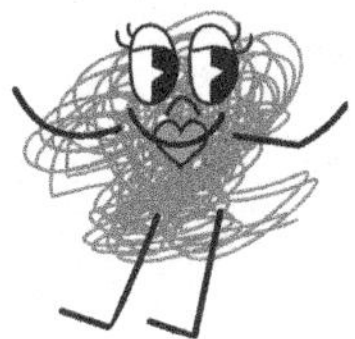	*Love/ Care*	Warm chest, gentle energy, wanting to help or protect	Is this something I can repeat or share? Can I enjoy it without rushing?
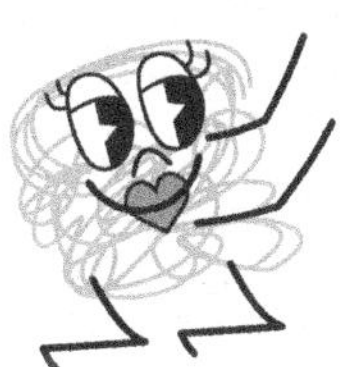	*Infatuation*	Obsessive thoughts, adrenaline, daydreaming, ignoring red flags	Am I seeing the full picture, or only the good parts? Is this feeling fading or growing?
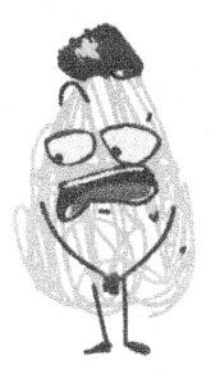	SHAME	Heat in face, avoiding eye contact, wanting to hide	Is this about a real mistake or someone else's opinion? What can I learn and move forward with?
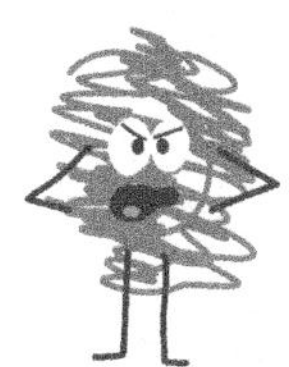	**Envy**	pain of sadness or anger, twist in your stomach, jealousy	What does this person have that I want? Why do I want it? Can I be happy for the other person?

EMOTIONAL STRENGTHS AND WEAKNESSES

Don't let your feelings run the show

Emotions are part of being human. They're like the notifications on your phone—telling you something's going on inside.

Anger gives you the energy and courage to stand up for yourself or others. However, it can also make you say or do things you later regret, pushing people away.

Fear can protect you by warning you of danger and making you cautious.It can stop you from trying new things or taking a healthy risk.

Joy can connect you to others and fill you with energy and hope.It can sometimes make you careless or not take a situation seriously enough.

Sadness

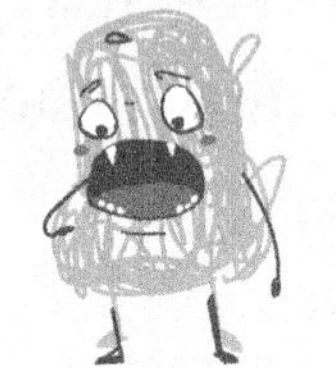

Sadness can let you know something is wrong and that you need comfort or to heal.It can make you feel helpless and stop you from trying to move forward.

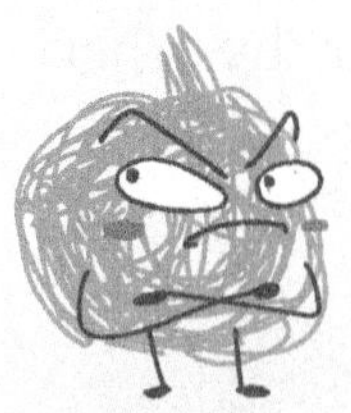

Envy can show you what you truly want and motivate you to work for it.It can lead to resentment and stop you from celebrating the success of others.

Confidence can give you the belief to try, even if you are afraid.It can make you overconfident and cause you to make a careless mistake.

STRESS-BUSTER WORD SEARCH

Find the words below that are all ways to help you manage stress.
The words can be found horizontally, vertically, or diagonally.

A	C	I	N	W	K	L	P	A	M	M	L
C	R	N	P	L	A	Y	L	B	R	E	A
C	R	E	A	T	I	V	I	T	Y	H	C
A	E	T	A	T	I	D	E	M	C	T	C
S	T	S	S	H	S	T	R	T	R	A	E
L	L	I	N	F	L	U	E	N	C	E	P
W	A	L	K	S	B	R	A	L	P	R	T
N	U	P	O	O	T	S	D	T	E	B	A
I	G	P	O	S	I	T	I	V	E	W	N
N	H	W	A	L	N	L	C	A	L	A	C
T	P	O	U	T	D	O	O	R	S	M	E

Hint: Some words are backwards

ACCEPTANCE	POSITIVE	LAUGH
OUTDOORS	SLEEP	PLAY
TALK	WALK	MEDITATE
BREATHE	STRETCH	CREATIVITY
READ	LISTEN	INFLUENCE

DECODE BEFORE YOU DECIDE

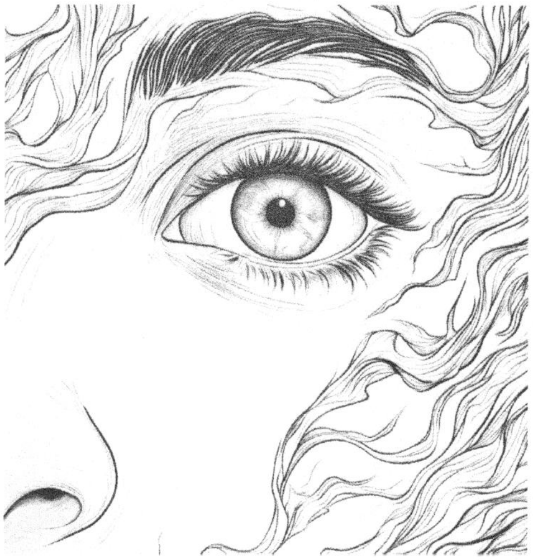

Think of a big choice you made in your life that wasn't the best
Which emotion was driving you?
Why was that emotion in control?

Think about a time when you acted before thinking. Write down what you might do differently next time.

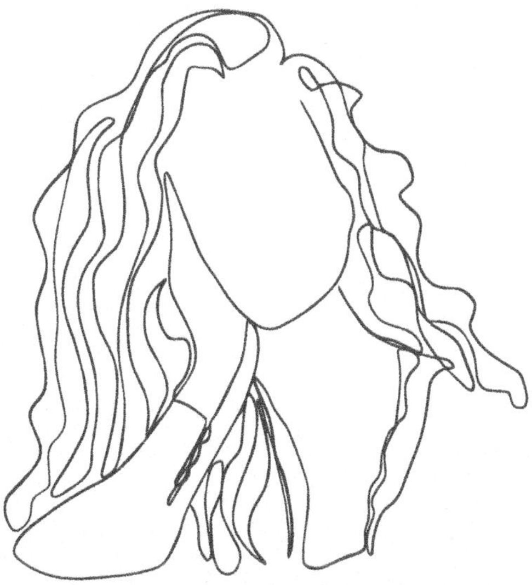

REGULATION STRATEGIES

Feeling stressed? Overstimulated? Frustrated? A mix of everything? Here are some quick activities you can do to regulate your emotions.

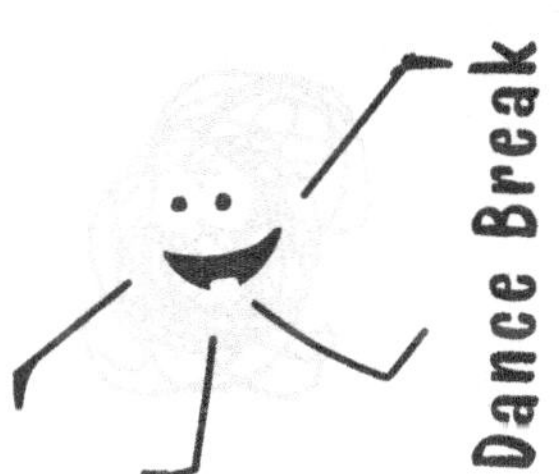

Dance Break

How?

Choose a song that helps you feel happy and energized. Dance it out! Go crazy and move to the music as you feel your body relax and your mind calm.

Why?

Taking a dance break helps regulate emotions by releasing endorphins and reducing stress, which can elevate mood and improve your emotional well being. The physical activity and rhythmic movement also provide an outlet for expressing and processing emotions.

Mindful Breathing

How?

Find a comfortable spot to sit with your back straight but relaxed and your hands on your lap or knees. Close your eyes and take a deep breath in through your nose. Count to 4. Hold your breath as you count to 4 again. Breathe out slowly and gently through your mouth while counting to 3. Continue this cycle until you feel calm and relaxed. stay present in the moment.

Why?

Mindful breathing helps regulate emotions by focusing attention on your breath, which calms your mind and body. It reduces stress and anxiety by slowing your breathing and helping you stay present in the moment.

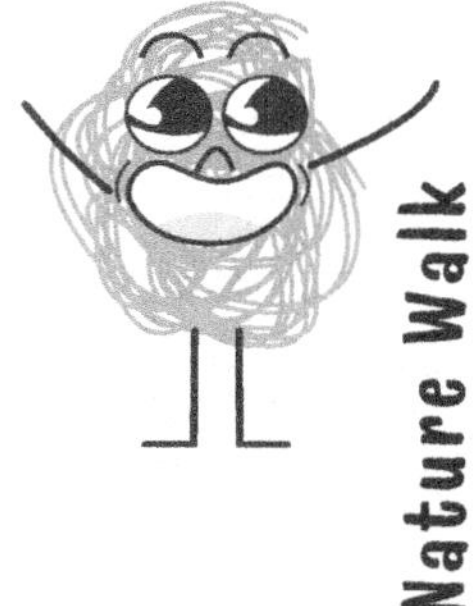

Nature Walk

How?

Find an area outside of your house or classroom that is safe to walk. As you walk, listen to the sounds you hear, what your smell, how the air feels on your skin, what the ground sounds like as you step, and how the leaves of the plants feel against your skin.

Why?

Going on a nature walk helps reduce stress and makes you feel calmer by connecting with the peaceful environment around you. Walking boosts your mood and energy by releasing chemicals in your brain that make you feel good.

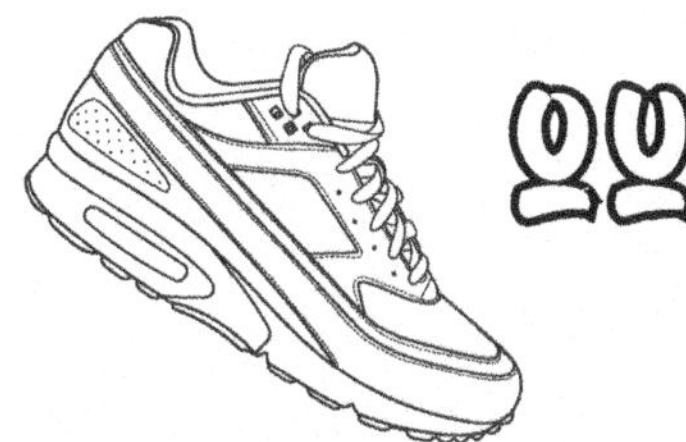

OUTSIDE INFLUENCES

The Battle of the Brands

Imagine you're walking through a mall with your best friend, Sammy. All week, Sammy has been obsessed with this new brand of sneakers called "Hyper Kicks." They're everywhere online—all the cool influencers are wearing them. Sammy says they're the only shoes that matter.

But as you pass the sneaker store, you see a display for "Comfy Clouds," a brand you've never heard of. You try them on. They're like walking on air. They also cost half as much as Hyper Kicks. You're super excited, but when you show Sammy, they just shrug. "They're not popular," Sammy says. "No one wears them."

Suddenly, your excitement fades. You start to feel embarrassed. You put the shoes back and leave the store, feeling confused. Even though your feet felt great and you know the price is better, you've been influenced by Sammy's opinion, which was influenced by a bunch of famous people online. Your own feelings were pushed aside by a feeling of wanting to fit in.

Reflect

What role did your emotions play in this story? How did your feeling of excitement change?

What emotion do you think Alex was feeling that made them say, "No one wears them?"

If you could go back to the store, what would you do or say differently?

WHAT EMOTIONS DRIVE YOU?

What emotions do you seek most often when looking for entertainment (social media, video games, art, or music)

1. ______________________________
2. ______________________________
3. ______________________________
4. ______________________________
5. ______________________________

When you are alone looking for a book, game, or song are there certain emotions you seek out more often then others? If so which ones? Why?

EMOTION IN ADVERTISING

"They know how you feel and they use it to get your attention, your trust, and your money."

Every day, we are bombarded with messages from ads, posts, and content from influencers on all sorts of social media platforms. Companies spend billions designing content to make us feel something. They all need us to watch, click, share, or buy and they use our feelings because research shows that when we feel something good or bad, we are more likely to do something. In other words, our emotions drive actions. And they need us to act.

Think about it

Sadness → makes us want comfort →
"buy something or watch something uplifting"

Excitement → makes us act quickly →
"buy now before it's gone"

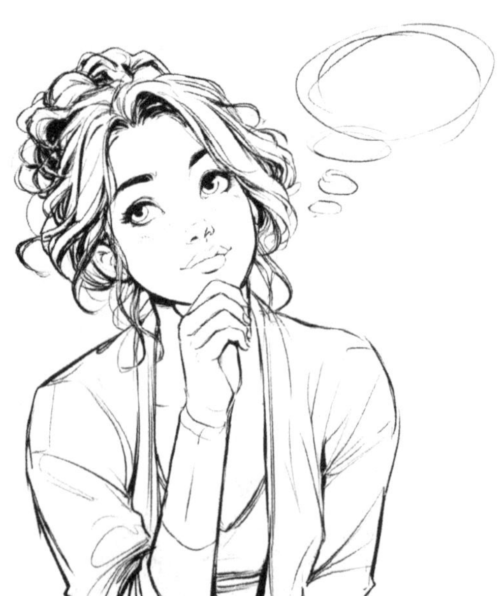

Fear → makes us want safety →
"listen to advice or follow someone who 'knows' the answer"

Belonging → makes us join in →
"follow trends so you fit in"

WANT TO BE AN INFLUENCER?

Follow the "Influencer Formula"

Use this page to create an ad for something you would like to promote through social media. Use the steps to guide you.

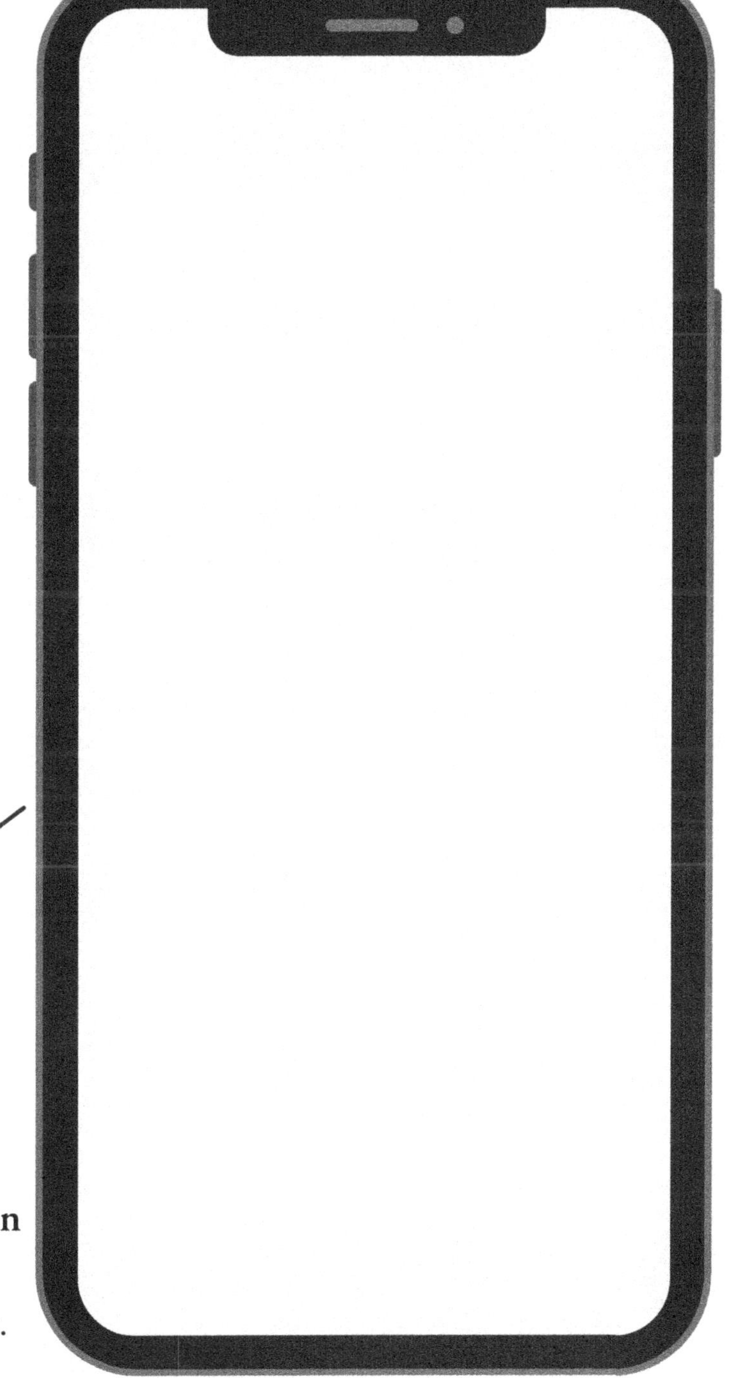

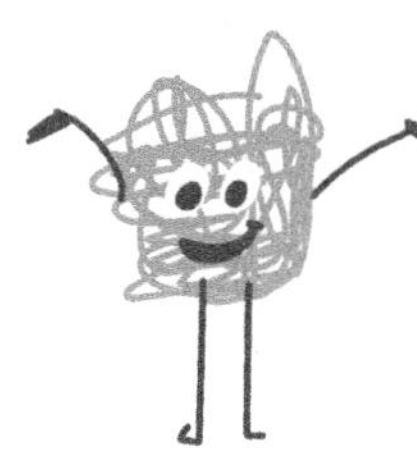

1. Trigger an Emotion
Think about music, colors, faces, words, stories.

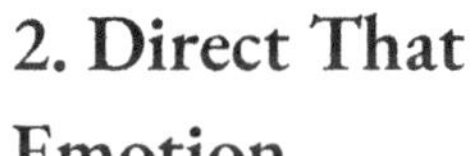

2. Direct That Emotion
"This is the solution to your problem" or "Join the fun!"

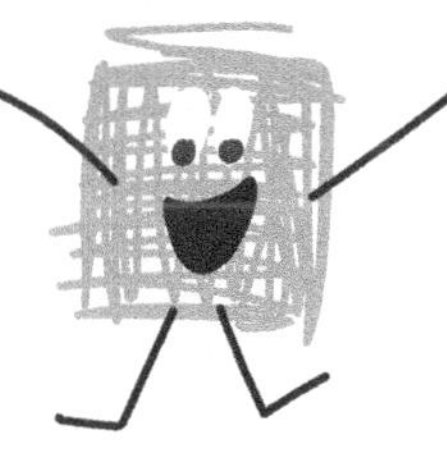

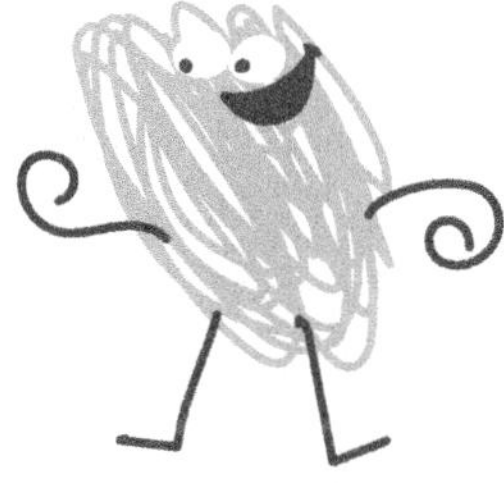

3. Call to Action
Buy it. Watch it. Share it. Follow it.

BE AN AD DETECTIVE

Find an ad, TikTok, or YouTube video you've seen recently that made you feel something.

What is the product or message?

____

____

____

____

____

____

Which emotion did it try to trigger?

(See page 56 for the list)

____

____

____

____

____

Did it work on you? Why?

____

____

____

____

____

____

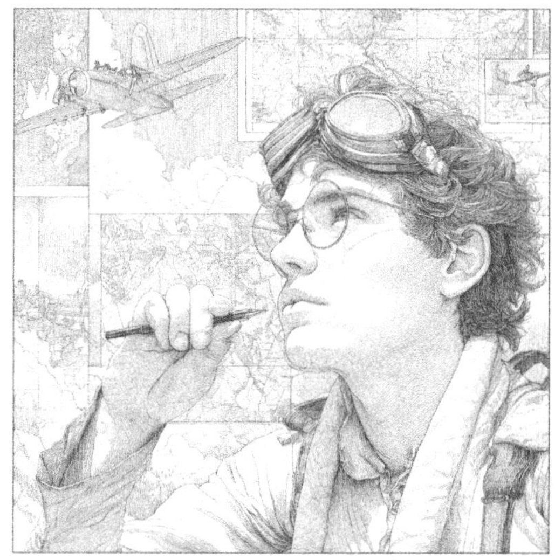

PRO TIP

Just because someone triggers an emotion doesn't mean you have to follow it.

Pause and ask:

Is this choice what I want—or what they want?

PART THREE:

BE AN INFLUENCER

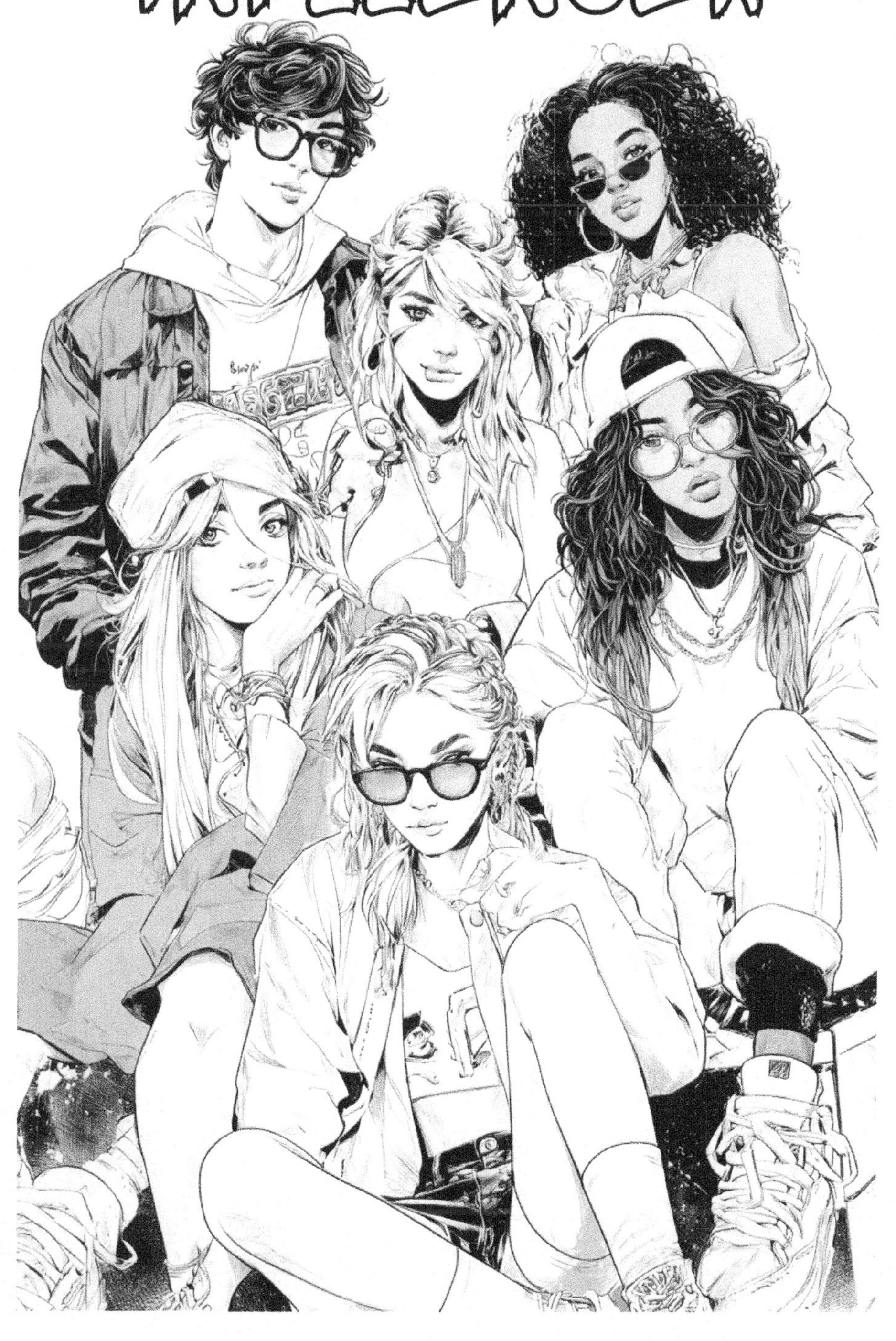

THE VLOGGER

Sienna's screen glowed as she watched. It was like looking through a portal into a world of perfect lives. The "EliteVlog," a channel featuring perfectly styled girls whose sponsors provided them with trips and an endless supply of clothes. Sienna watched excitedly as the vloggers made their way through the mall. The girls laughed, then they whispered, "Watch this."

Looking right into the camera, they grinned as they snuck snacks into their bags.

Sienna's heart dropped. This had to be a stunt.

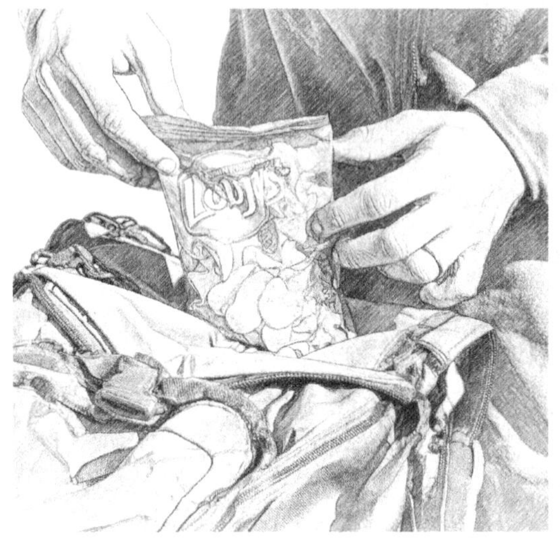

But the next week, it happened again. This was no stunt. They were taking whatever they wanted and making it look so fun. At first, Sienna thought it was dishonest, but they just made it look so exciting. Nothing exciting ever happened to Sienna. Maybe this is why they were influencers and she was just the influenced.

A voice, soft as a shadow, whispered in her ear, "Why watch when you can do?" it asked. Sienna's palms sweated. Maybe she just needed to throw caution to the wind. Her heart pounded. She thought of the likes, the comments, the rush. All she had to do was hide a phone and head to the local store--no one was ever watching!

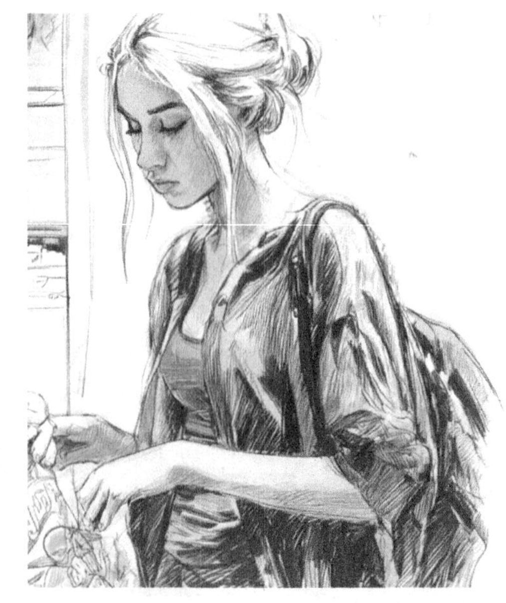

Her hands trembled as she took the headphones from the shelf and tucked them into her sleeve. Her cheeks felt hot, her mind raced, and her feet wobbled as she tried to act perfectly normal as she left the store.

The second she walked in her front door, she felt a shame was hotter than any spotlight. Her mom took one look at her flushed cheeks and the interrogation began. Soon her phone was gone and all other technology too. But it wasn't the consequence, not even having to apologize to the store owner, that ate at her;

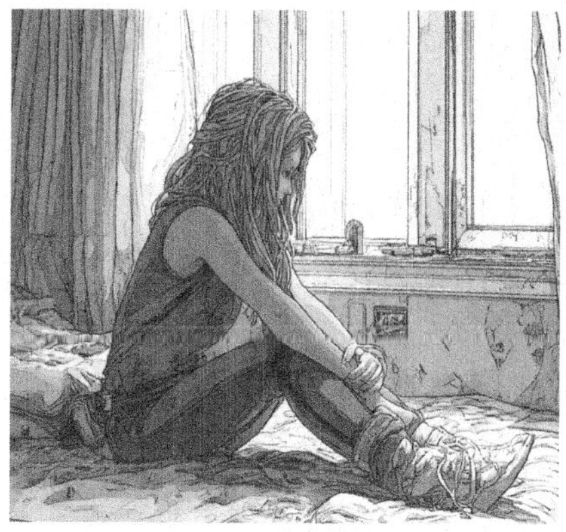

it was the way her mom refused to look her in the eye; the way the house felt sour and bitter all at the same time; and the way she hated herself for what she'd done. She'd just wanted to feel cool, but now she's empty, alone, and so ashamed.

Imagine that you are Sienna. What would you have done in this situation?

____

____

____

____

____

____

____

____

____

____

____

____

____

THE GAMER

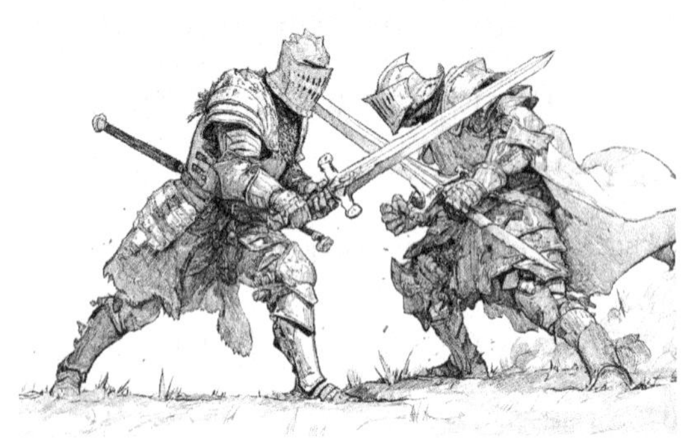

The digital stadium roared. Leo's clenched his controller as his avatar, a fiery knight, stood ready. King Midas, his commander, took a deep breath and gave the order: “Attack the weak one. No mercy." The target was clear. They were turning on one of their own. And that knight just happened to be Leo’s real-life friend from school, Jaiden.

Leo felt his hands freeze. He couldn’t kill Jaiden. They had a pact to help each other. Besides they were supposed to be on the same team! But King Midas's voice echoed in his headphones. “Finish him or we’ll finish you! The entire company filled with cheers as they pounded the their swords to their shields. “Finish him,” they chanted.

Leo's finger hovered over the attack button, his mind a battlefield. And then he did it. He launched the final, decisive blow. Jaiden’s knight fell to the ground, and the screen flashed "Victory." The company cheered, but Leo did not feel victorious. He closed his eyes and tried to forget. Maybe, it would be okay. Maybe, Jaiden would understand.

The next day when Leo say Jaiden, he lifted his hand in a wave and walked toward him, calling his name. Jaiden took one look at Leo, and turn away. “Jaiden, come back,” Leo called after him. Jaiden walked faster. Leo didn’t blame him. He’d broken their pact and now he had to face the consequence: a broken friendship for a fleeting, virtual win.

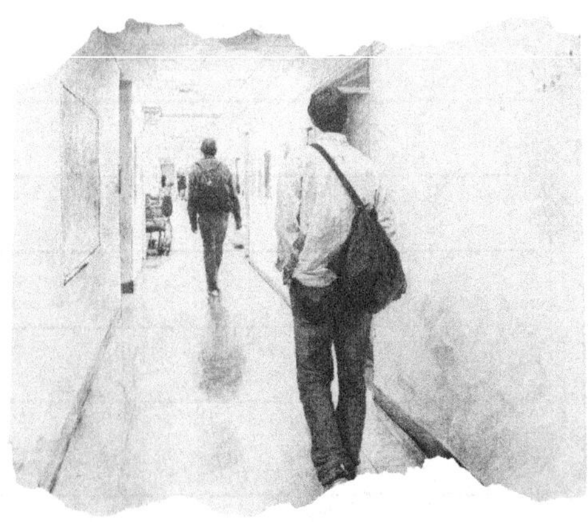

THE GROUP CHAT

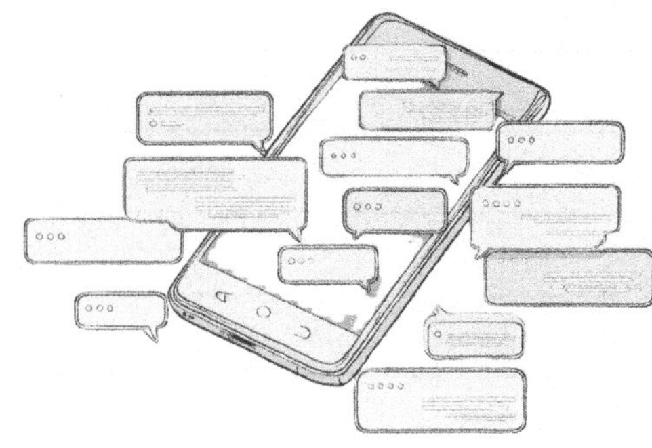

Alex's phone buzzed. It was the group chat again with their constant stream of memes and gossip. A new message read: "Have you seen what Maria is wearing today?" It was followed by a picture, taken from a distance, and a series of laughing emojis. Within minutes, a wave of mean comments followed. Everyone in the group had responded. Everyone except Maria and of course Alex, who's thumb was frozen.

Maria was kind and shy. Had they forgotten she was in the chat? A feeling of sickness bubbled up. Alex's fingers pressed into the screen, then stopped. The fear of being the next target grew. Alex didn't want to be left out, or worse kicked out. But adding to it would be wrong. Alex didn't make fun of people, especially not nice people. The response would be to do nothing, which felt good until Maria's name exited the chat. It was a quiet exit with no goodbye, but to Alex it was louder that if she had messaged with all caps in bold.

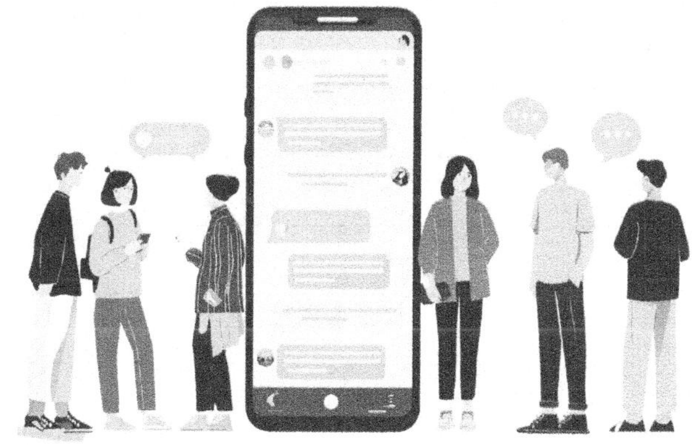

The next morning, when Maria walked past Alex, her eyes were red. Her head hung low, and her lips pursed tight. Alex wanted to say hello, to say her outfit was cute, but nothing she could say now would make amends for the sting of yesterday's silence. Alex had been a coward. She'd chosen to stand on the side of cruelty instead of compassion. Her phone buzzed. It was the group chat. Suddenly, nothing they said mattered. The memes, jokes, and supposed friends were as filtered as an Instagram post. Alex wanted real friends, not hollow screens of scorn. "Maria, wait," Alex said, chasing her down.

Reflect and Connect

Think about the stories you read. Why was it difficult for the characters to defend their friends?

Have you ever had a time when you should have stood up for someone and didn't?

Have you ever had someone stand up for you or not stand up for you? What did it feel like?

DANGEROUS MEDIA

The Rise and Fall of "The Trickster"

There's this incredibly popular YouTuber, let's call him "The Trickster." Famous for doing crazy stunts with his friends and family. Funny and original his videos pulled millions of views. But over time, each video got more extreme. His pranks went from surprising to dangerous.

Your friend, Leo, is OBSESSED with The Trickster. He's even started to copy his pranks on people at school. You try to tell Leo that what he's doing is wrong, but he says, "It's just a joke! People love it. Trickster gets millions of view."

It's all whatever until one day, Leo's prank on the new kid goes too far. Pretty soon parents, the principal, and event the police are involved. Luckily the new kid is okay, but he switches schools. Leo gets suspended and then sent away to a school for troubled kids. Now one of your best friends is gone and even though you warned Leo not to prank people, everyone thinks you were in on it.

How did The Trickster's videos influence Leo's actions and emotions?

____

____

What do you think the stakes are of not checking bad influences in your life?

____

____

How can you tell the difference between a funny, harmless video and one that might lead to bad decisions?

____

____

____

Why do you think some people, like Leo, are so influenced by what's popular online?

____

____

____

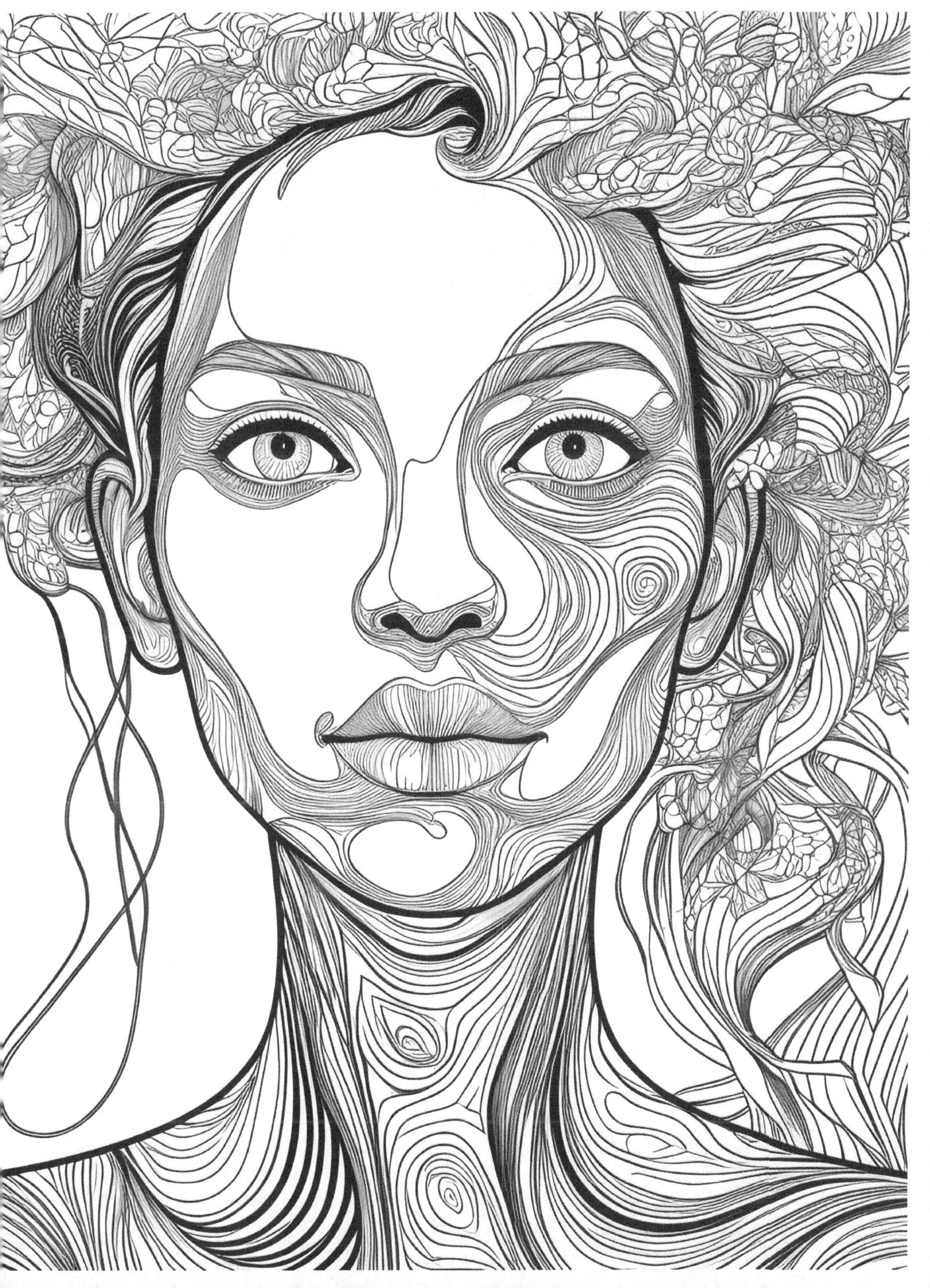

THE POWER OF SMALL THINGS

The biggest changes come from the smallest actions.

You have the power to influence your own life.

We often think that to be an influencer, we have to do one huge, amazing thing. But as James Clear explains in his book, Atomic Habits, the small things we do every single day have the biggest impact.

The "Atomic Habit" Idea

Think of a small habit, like making your bed. It seems tiny, but it starts a chain reaction of positive actions. You've already accomplished one thing, so you're more likely to do another. Over time, these small actions compound into big changes.*

Write a tiny habit you can start today above the first domino. Imagine that each domino contains a tiny habit that will lead to one big change. Above the final domino, write down a big goal that this tiny habit could lead to over time.

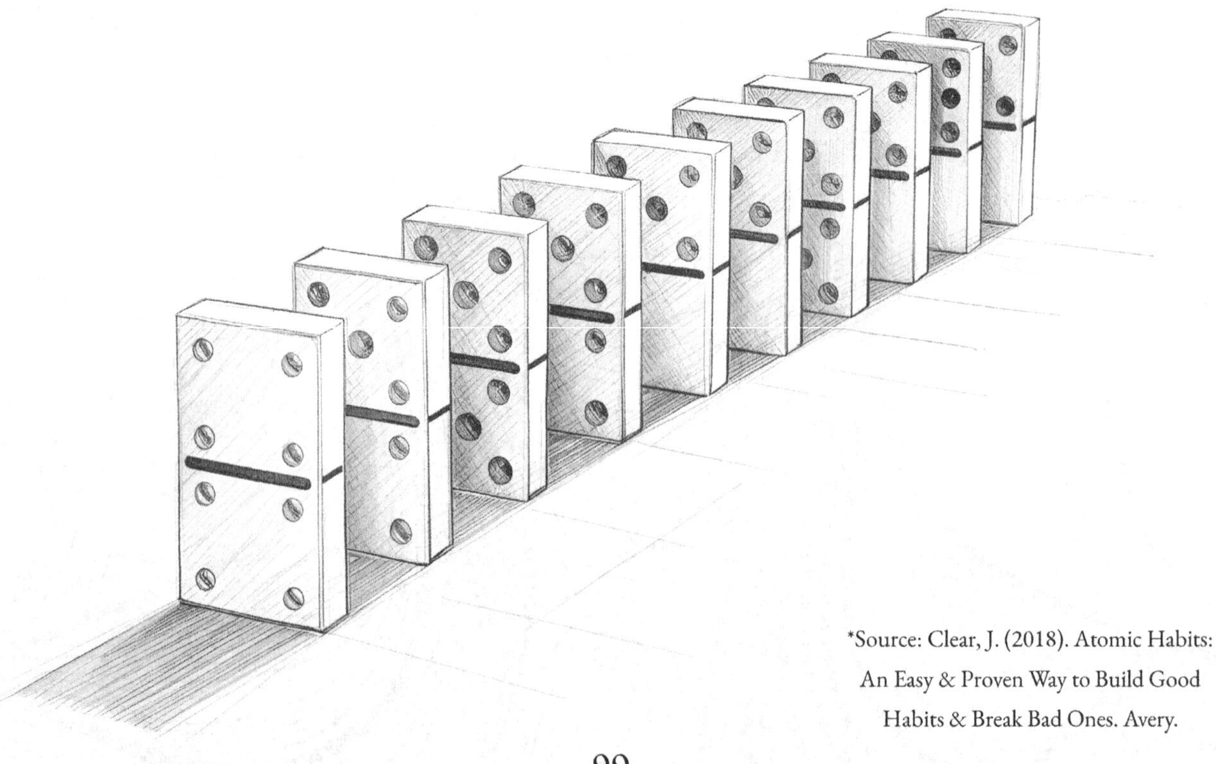

*Source: Clear, J. (2018). Atomic Habits: An Easy & Proven Way to Build Good Habits & Break Bad Ones. Avery.

WHAT SHOULD YOU CHANGE?

The biggest changes come from the smallest actions.

You have the power to influence your own life.

Look at the circle below. Think about your life.

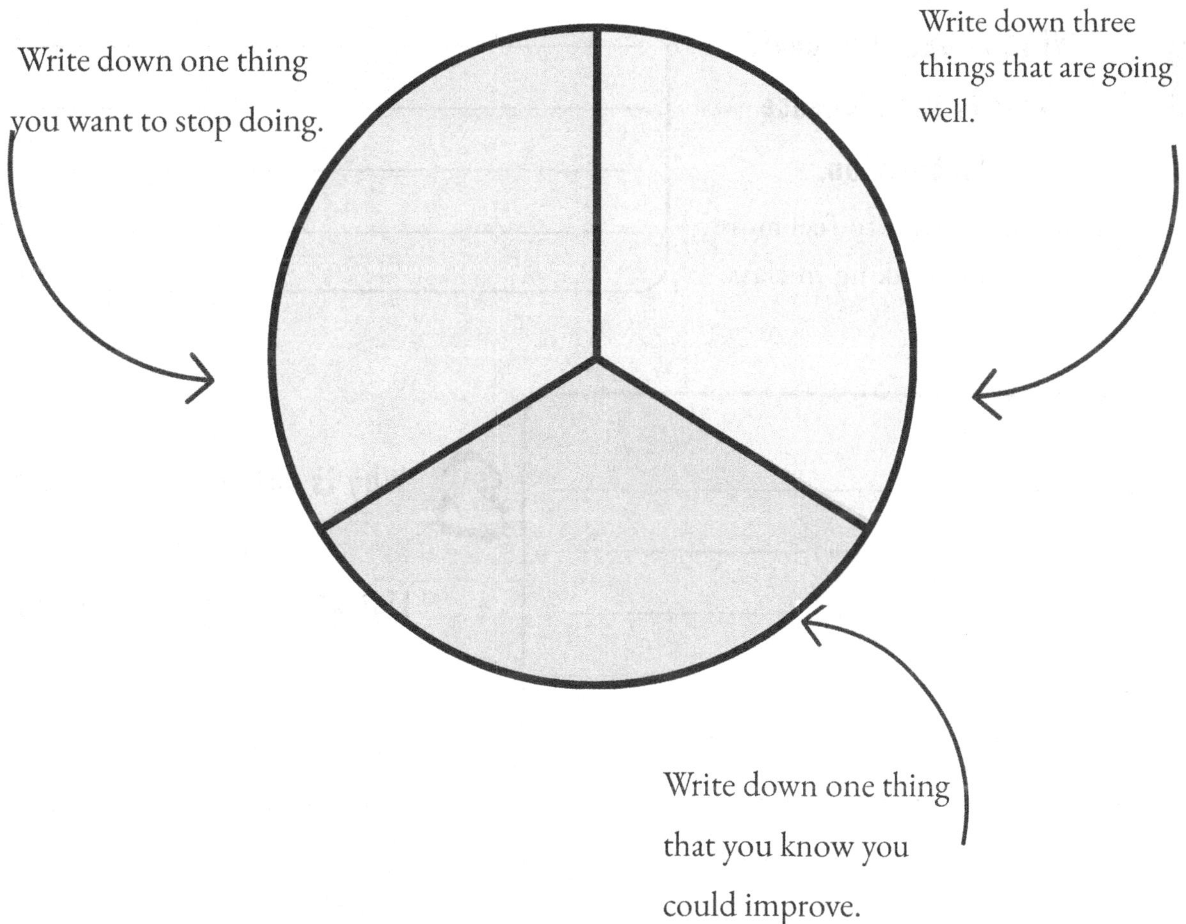

Choose just ONE small change you can make this week. Write it down here.

Explain how this small change will have a positive influence on your life.

INFLUENCER GOALS

Becoming a better influencer starts with you.
When you have goals for yourself, you influence your own life.
Follow these steps to create your influencer goals.

1 **What is your BIG goal? This is the ultimate destination.**

Example: I want to feel more confident speaking in class.

2 **Why is this goal important to you? List at least three reasons.**

Example:

1. I have good ideas I want to share.
2. I want to feel less nervous.
3. I want to be a leader in my group.

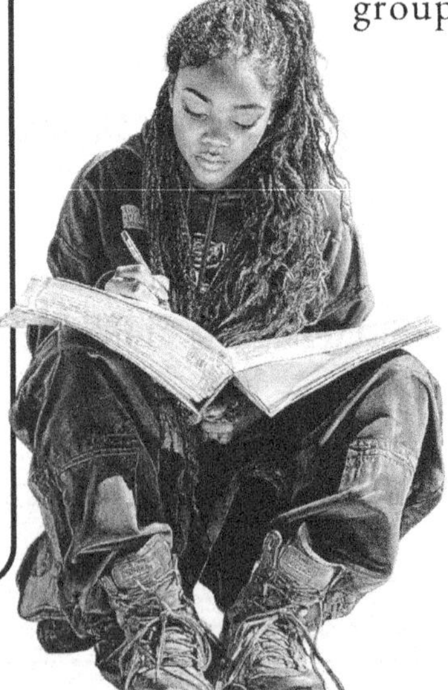

3 Break it down into small steps. List three steps you can take to reach your goal.

Example:

Practice speaking to my family at the dinner table.

Write down one thing I want to say in class each day.

Raise my hand to ask one question per week.

4 Action Plan.

What is the first small step you will take, and when will you do it?

5 Check-in and Celebrate!

After a week, reflect on your progress.

Did you meet your first goal? What can you do to celebrate your effort?

HOW DO YOU COMMUNICATE?

Read each scenario on the following page.

Draw a picture or symbol next to the letter you most agree with. At the end, count the drawings by each letter to determine which type of communicator you are.

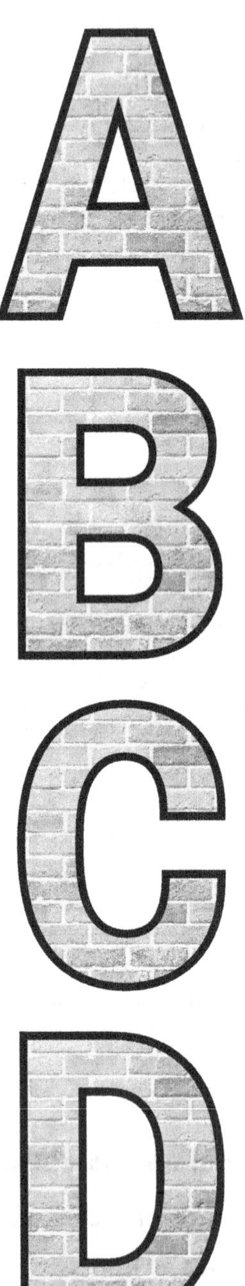

"The biggest communication problem is that we do not listen to understand. We listen to reply."

iCleave

COMMUNICATION STYLE QUIZ

1 **When you're faced with a tough decision, you usually:**

a) Trust your gut and make a choice that feels right for you, even if it's not popular.
b) Carefully weigh all the options, considering the pros and cons before acting.
c) Ask for advice from people you trust, valuing their perspective before deciding.
d) Think about the impact your decision will have on others and choose the option that will best serve the group.

2 **When you're trying to share an idea, you focus on:**

a) Expressing yourself with passion and authenticity, letting your enthusiasm lead the way.
b) Organizing your thoughts logically, using clear and precise language to get your point across.
c) Listening to others first to understand their needs and tailor your message to them.
d) Building consensus and finding a common ground where everyone feels heard and included.

3 **In a conflict, your first instinct is to:**

a) Speak up honestly about how you feel, even if it's uncomfortable.
b) Step back to process your emotions and analyze the situation before responding.
c) Try to understand the other person's point of view and find a way to empathize.
d) Focus on de-escalating the tension and finding a solution that works for everyone involved.

4 **The communication style you most admire in others is:**

a) Someone who is brave enough to share their unique story, even if it's messy.
b) Someone who is thoughtful and articulate, always having a well-researched opinion.
c) Someone who is a great listener and can connect with people on a deep level.
d) Someone who is a natural leader and can bring different people together for a common cause.

5 **You feel your message is most powerful when it:**

a) Sparks a strong emotional response in others and inspires them to take action.
b) Is backed by facts and data, proving your point beyond a doubt.
c) Creates a feeling of community and connection among people.
d) Leads to a tangible, positive change in your group or community.

WHAT KIND OF COMMUNICATOR ARE YOU?

Your Influencer Communication Style

Count up your answers to find your primary communication style and read about its strengths and weaknesses below.

THE STORY TELLER

mostly

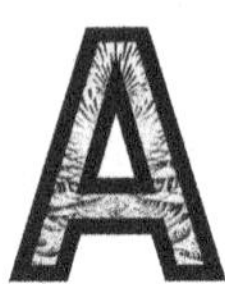

As a natural storyteller, you communicate with authentic and raw passion. You inspire others by showing your vulnerabilities and leading with your heart. Your communication is often unfiltered and driven by strong emotions, which makes it exciting. It also creates deep, personal connection with their audience.

STRENGTHS

- **Authenticity**- You are true to your own communication style and self.
- **Courage** You inspire others through your raw, unfiltered passion.
- **Natural storyteller**- You aren't afraid to show your vulnerabilities, which builds a strong emotional connection with your audience.

WEAKNESSES

- **Impulsive**- Your strong emotions can occasionally lead to communication that is not well-thought-out. This means it can be inaccurate or even hurt people's feelings
- **Bias**- As a passionate storyteller, you can sometimes get lost in the story and only tell the facts that highlight the moral or perspective you are highlighting, which can create a bias.

EXPERT

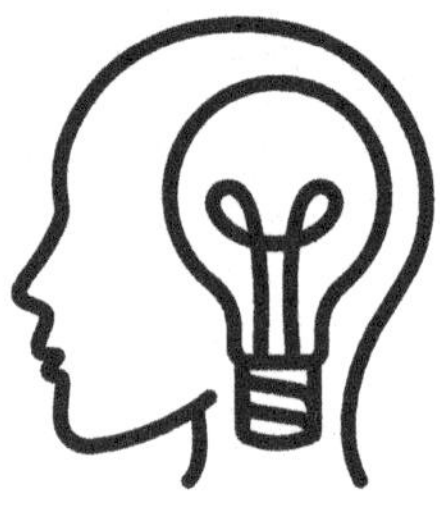

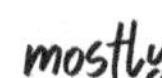

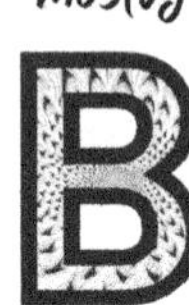

Experts communicate with clarity, precision, and purpose. Your words are backed by data and careful research, making your arguments logical and compelling. You are valued for your ability to explain complex ideas and provide well-reasoned, intellectual insights.

STRENGTHS

- **Direct:** Your communication style is clear, logical, and evidence-based. You save time and make sure that people understand what you are saying.
- **Efficient:** You are valued for your ability to analyze complex topics and present information in a way that is easy to understand. You are purposeful with every word.

WEAKNESSES

- **Detached:** You may struggle to connect on an emotional level and can sometimes be seen as detached or overly formal.
- **Narrowly focused:** You may struggle to see other people's perspective or open the communication for creative ideas and expression.

COMMUNITY BUILDER

mostly C

As a Community Builder you are all about empathy and connection. You are exceptional listeners who prioritize making others feel seen and heard. You excel at building a sense of belonging and fostering strong, meaningful relationships. Your goal is to unite people and create a space where everyone feels valued.

STRENGTHS

- **Dependable:** You are always there, providing consistent support and presence in others' lives.
- **Listener:** You are a great listener who offers thoughtful and compassionate advice.
- **Champion:** You support others and will cheer for them even when their goals are different from your own.

WEAKNESSES

- **Overcommitted:** You may struggle to say no, taking on too much responsibility for your friends and potentially neglecting your own needs.
- **Avoidant:** You may prioritize harmony over honesty, sometimes avoiding difficult conversations to prevent conflict.

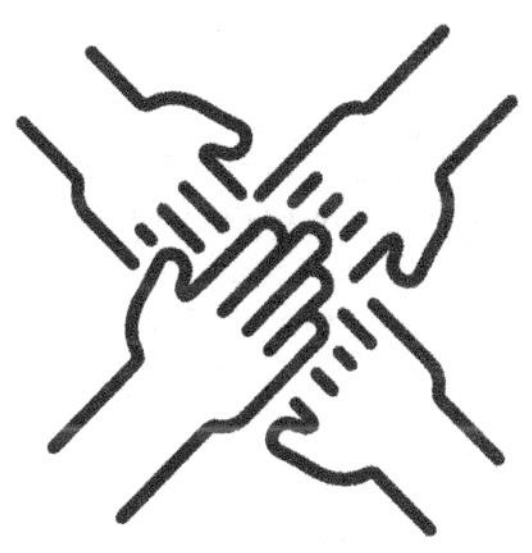

COLLABORATOR

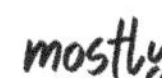

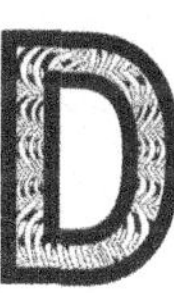

You are a skilled diplomat and natural leader. You focus on teamwork and finding common ground. You are a master at de-escalating conflict and bringing diverse groups together to achieve a shared goal.

STRENGTHS

- **Motivate:** You are a gifted communicator who knows how to unite people and make them feel excited to share in a common goal.
- **Supportive:** Your communication style is focused on finding common ground, fostering teamwork, and creating positive change. You excel at motivating groups and leading projects to success.

WEAKNESSES

- **Overwhelmed:** Your ability to motivate and unite people can cause you to have too many projects and people who want your attention, leading you to feel overwhelmed
- **Focus:** You may lose your sense of self and direction when you are trying to make everyone happy.

CONVERSATION BREAKDOWN

Think about a recent conversation you had with someone else that didn't go as well as you hoped it would. Maybe you felt misunderstood or the other person seemed frustrated.

Whas was the main goal of the conversation?

Consider the description of your communication style on the last two pages as you answer the following questions.

Where did your natural tendencies help the conversation?

Where did your natural tendencies hurt the conversation?

Knowing your style now, what is one thing you could have done differently?

STYLE SWAP DISCUSSION

Find a friend or partner who also took the communication styles quiz. Do not reveal your results to one another.

My friend thinks my communication style is

____

I think my friend's communication style is

____

My communication style is actually...

____

My friend's communication style is actually...

____

Our #1 communication strength is...

____

Our #1 communication challenge is...

____

One thing we can work on to be better communicators with each other.

____

____

____

____

COMMUNICATE EFFECTIVELY

Being a good communicator is a superpower. It helps you understand others and make yourself understood. Here are three ways you can be a better communicator.

"I Feel" Statements

When you use "I Feel" statements, you focus on your own emotions instead of blaming others. This helps others understand you better.

Change the following "You" statements to "I Feel" Statements.

You make me so mad when you don't listen!	I feel frustrated when I'm not being listened to.
You never let me talk.	______________________
You're so annoying when you interrupt.	______________________

The Active Listener

When you use "I Feel" statements, you focus on your own emotions instead of blaming others. This helps others understand you better.

Practice this with a friend:

One person talks for two minutes about their day. The other person can only listen. After two minutes, the listener has to summarize what the person said and how they felt. Then you switch.

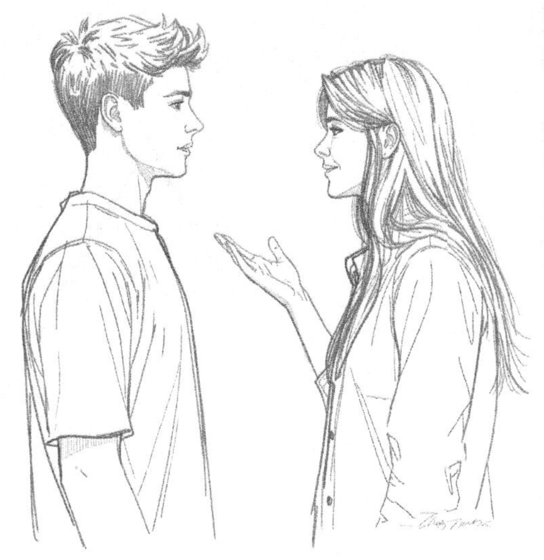

An active listener doesn't just hear words; they hear feelings. They listen with their eyes, ears, and heart.

Non-Verbal Cues

Communication is not just about words. It's about body language, tone of voice, and facial expressions.

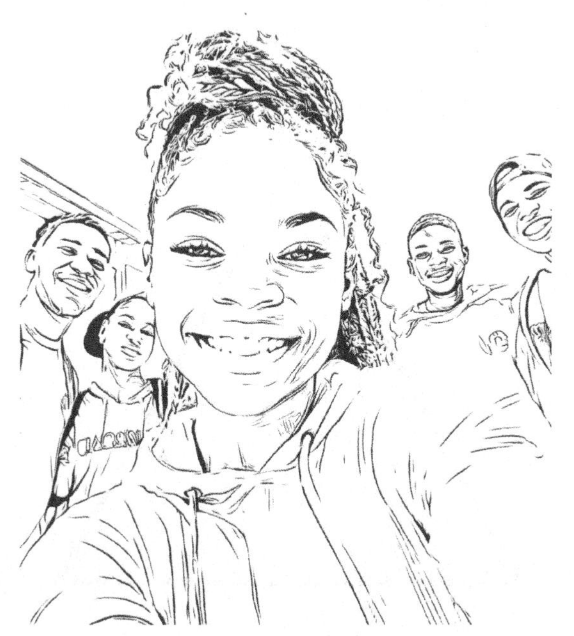

Act out these emotions for a friend or family member without saying a word. See if they can guess how you're feeling.

Annoyed

Excited

Confused

Tired

Proud

SKETCH BREAK

What can you draw starting with the shapes?

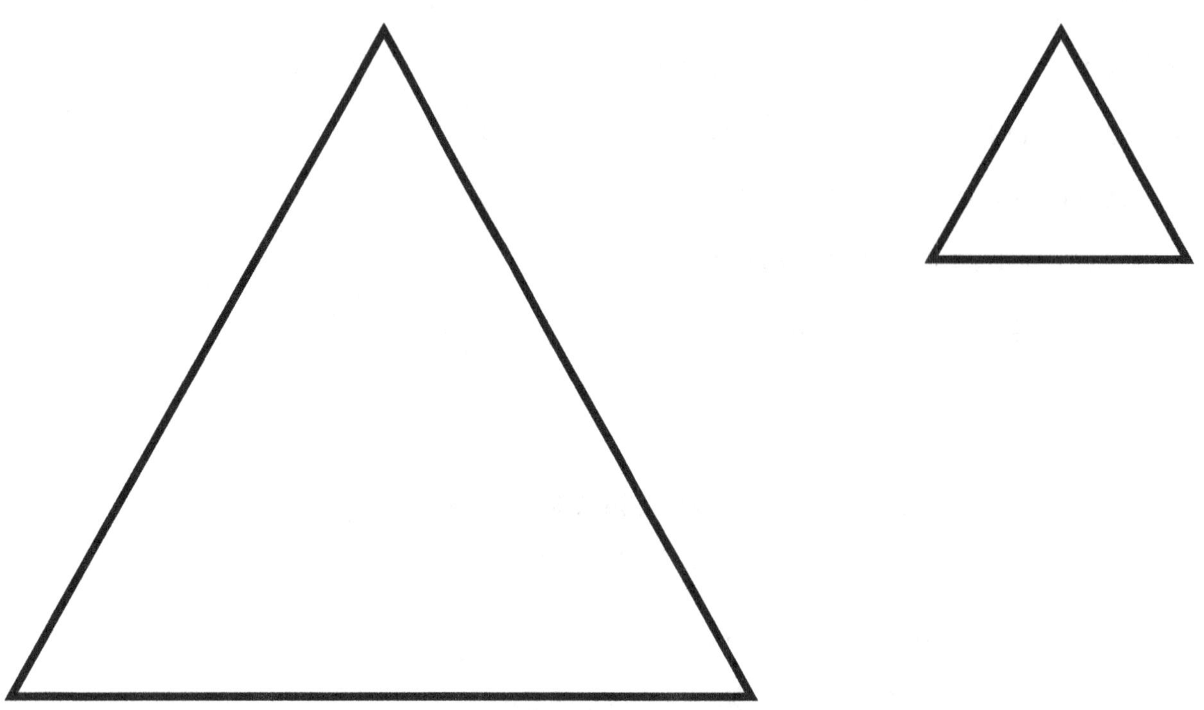

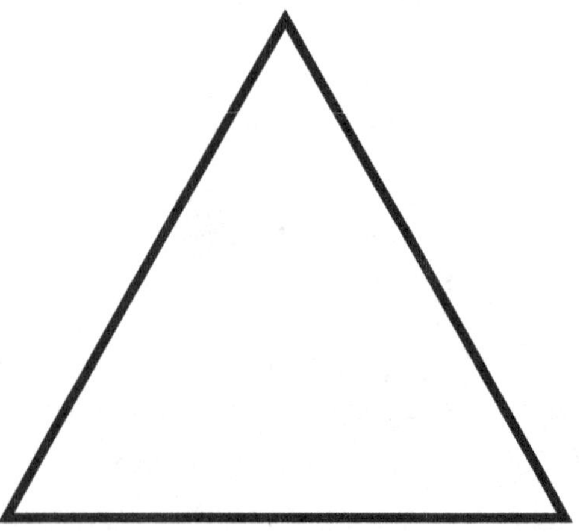

INCREASE YOUR INFLUENCE

Imagine your life is a song. Some parts are fast, while some are slow. The tempo and timing of your actions are everything. Knowing when to act and when to wait can make a huge difference in how much influence you have over your own life.

The Two-Minute Rule

Think of a situation where you felt rushed and made a bad decision. Maybe you said something in a group chat during an argument that you later regretted or responded rudely to someone.

Now, think about what might have happened if you had **waited just two minutes** before you responded. You could have cooled down, thought about what to say, or decided not to respond at all. The two-minute pause gives you back your influence over your own actions and emotions.

The Pause Challenge

For the rest of the day, when you feel angry, rushed, or frustrated, take a two-minute pause before you act.

Then reflect on what happened. Did the pause help?

My name is ______________ and I am an influencer.

I will use my voice to ______________

__________________________.

I stand for ____________________

__________________________.

I believe that my influence can

____

Signature:

INFLUENCER MANIFESTO

A manifesto is a public declaration of your intentions, values, and vision. It's a way of telling the world—and yourself—what you stand for. Think of it as a personal mission statement for your life. By writing your own manifesto, you're claiming your power to influence the world for good. Companies, governments, and indiviuals use a manifesto as a creed to live by, a statement of your values and purpose.

THE RIPPLE EFFECT

Writing down a specific, positive action you could take, like "compliment a classmate." Draw out the potential "ripple effect" of that single action.

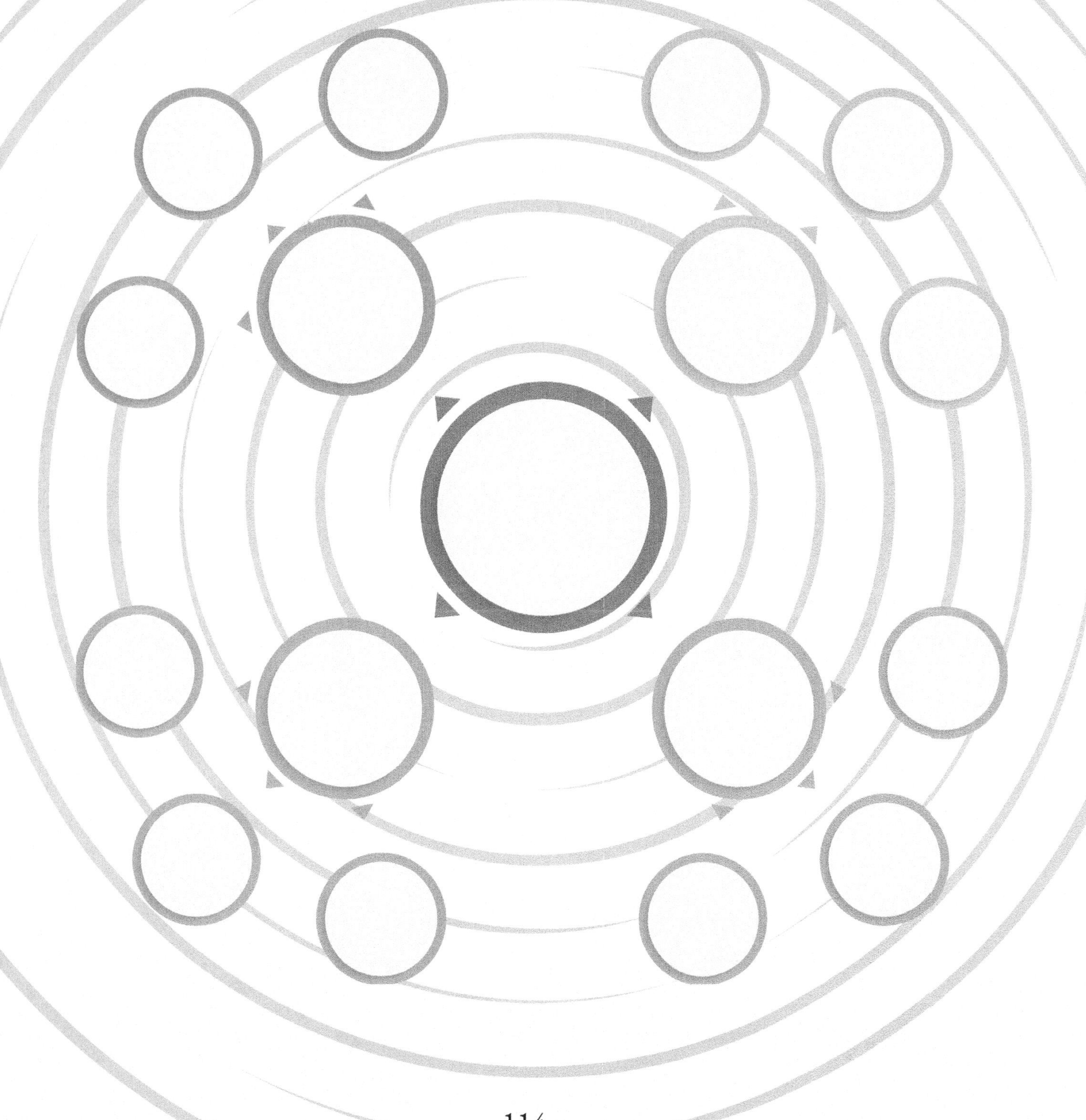

MY INFLUENCER PROJECT

Now it's time to put what you've learned into action!

You have the power to create a positive change in your community.

Your task is to create a small influencer project. It can be a social media campaign or a community effort. The goal is to use your influence for good. Here are some ideas:

- Create a social media account that shares positive stories and art.
- Organize a food or book drive at your school.
- Make a YouTube video series that teaches a skill you are good at, like drawing or coding.

Identify your audience.

Who do you want to influence?

____

____

____

____

____

____

How will you get noticed?

How will you use your talents to get people to pay attention?

____

____

____

____

____

____

What is your message?

What is the one big idea you want people to get?

____

____

____

____

Present your project idea to your class or a trusted adult.

Show them how you'll use what you've learned to be a positive influencer.

INFLUENCE TIME CAPSULE

A time capsule is a way to "send a letter to your future self."
Follow the steps to create a time capsule for yourself. This capsule will help you capture who you are today, what influences you most, and the mark you hope to leave on the world.

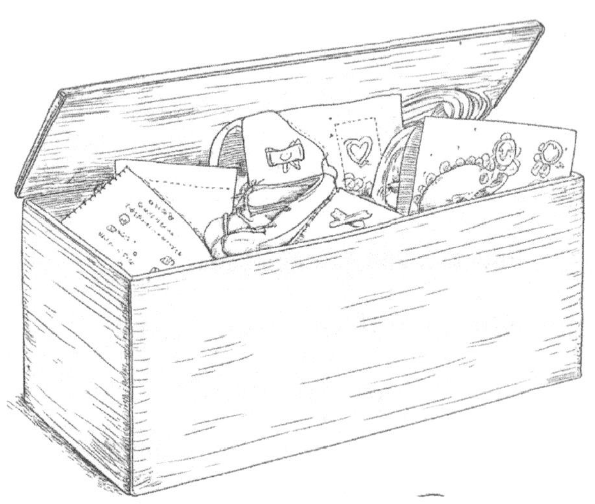

Select a container

Use a shoebox, tin, jar, or any sturdy container.
Decorate the outside with words or symbols that represent influence to you.

Reflect and write

Use the next page to write a letter to your future self about who influences you positively right now.

Consider who influences you and what impact you hope to have on the people around you.

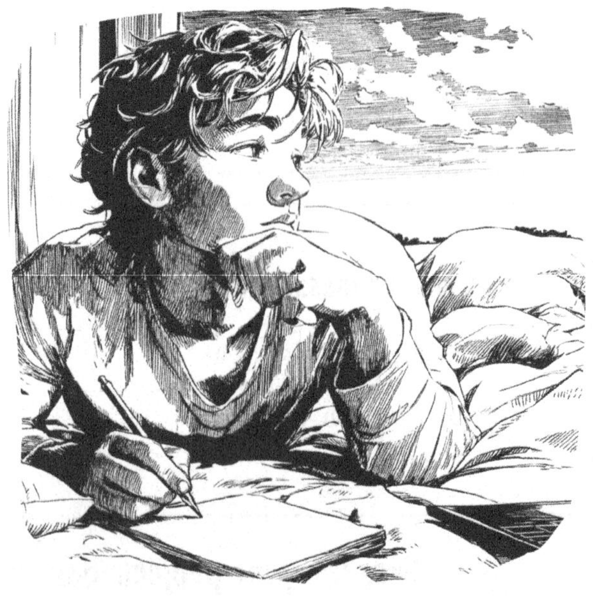

LETTER TO MY FUTURE SELF

Use the questions below to guide your letter to your future self that you can include in your time capsule.

1. Who influences you? What do they do that makes them a good influence? How do they shape the way you think, act, or feel?
2. How do you hope the influence the world around you?
3. What do you hope people will say about your impact?

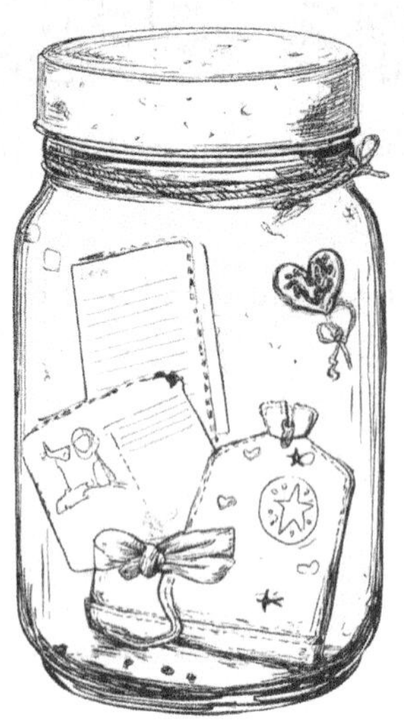

Collect your artifacts

Add meaningful items (some suggestions are below)

Line it with paper or fabric if you want it to feel special.

Put your chosen items and writings inside.

What Should I Include in My Time Capsule?

A letter to your future self

A photo of someone who influences you (or a drawing)

A small object that symbolizes growth (e.g., leaf, stone, or charm)

A page of your hopes, dreams, or goals

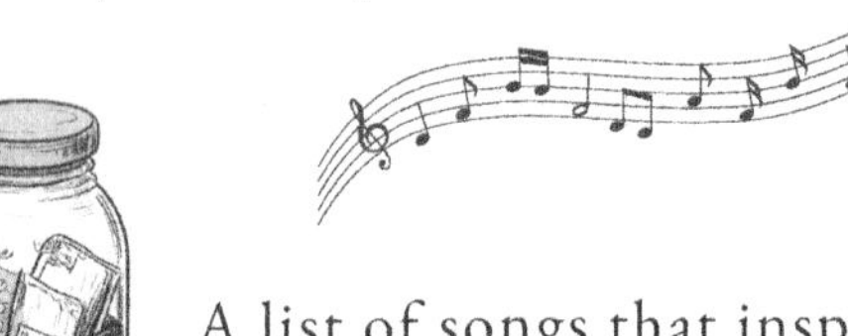

A list of songs that inspire you right now

A favorite quote, book passage, or saying that guides you

A doodle, poem, or short story about influence

Words of advice to your future self

A list of ways you want to influence the world positively

**This capsule isn't just about storing objects – it's about capturing your influence today and imagining the influence you will grow into.
When you open it in the future, you'll see how far you've come and how your vision of positive influence has unfolded.**

Seal and Store

Seal it securely with tape, string, or ribbon. You may cut and use the sign below to label your time capsule.

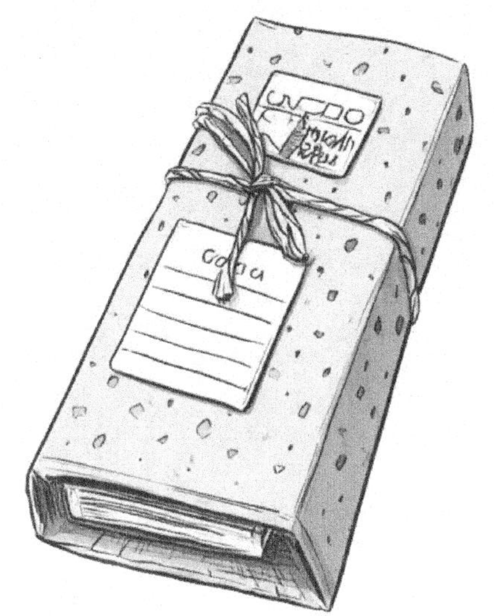

Store it somewhere safe but hidden, such as under your bed, in your closet, inside a drawer, or with a trusted adult who will remind you in the future.

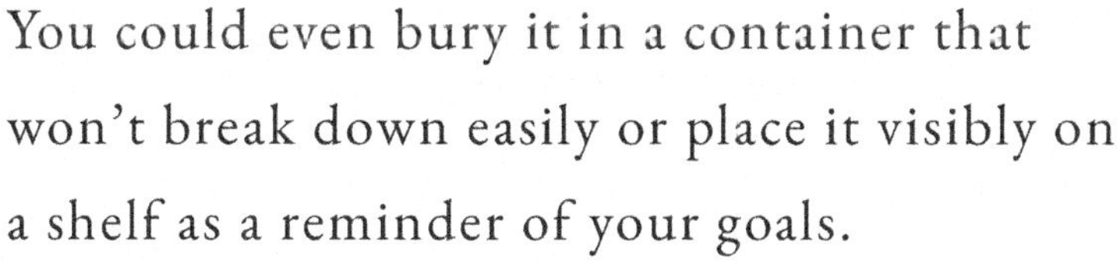

You could even bury it in a container that won't break down easily or place it visibly on a shelf as a reminder of your goals.

INFLUENCER TIME CAPSULE

Do not open until

____

Made in the USA
Coppell, TX
15 December 2025